DRUG-FREE PAIN RELIEF

A practical self-help guide to drug-free methods of pain relief using acupressure, transcutaneous nerve stimulation and psychological methods.

DRUG-FREE PAIN RELIEF
The Natural Way

by

George Lewith
M.A., M.R.C.G.P., M.R.C.P.
and
Sandra Horn
B.Tech. (Hons. Psych.), Dip. Clin. Psych.

THORSONS

THORSONS PUBLISHING GROUP
Wellingborough, Northamptonshire
Rochester, Vermont

First published 1987

© GEORGE LEWITH AND SANDRA HORN 1987

British Library Cataloguing in Publication Data

Lewith, George
   Pain relief: a self-help guide to drug-free methods.
   1. Analgesia
   I. Title   II. Horn, Sandra
   616'.0472   RB127

   ISBN 0-7225-1338-0

Printed and bound in Great Britain

Contents

Introduction

This book is divided into three sections. The first section will give you some general ideas about pain, what may cause it and how it is transmitted and processed by the body and in particular the nervous system.

The second section deals with two physical methods that you can use to treat your own pain. The first is acupressure, which involves the manual massage of acupuncture points, and the second is transcutaneous nerve stimulation (TNS); this involves using a small, cheap, battery-operated electric stimulator over the relevant acupuncture points. The exact nature of these techniques is described in some detail and simple but very specific instructions are given on how exactly to use these two treatments. Chapter 6 is devoted to a detailed discussion of some common painful conditions that can be treated with acupressure and TNS; the illnesses are listed along with specific instructions and illustrations about the best approach for each complaint. Chapter 6 can therefore be used as a manual for treatment. It is, however, very important that those wishing to use either acupressure or TNS should first read the chapters discussing the best way to use these techniques, before going on to the chapter that describes the treatment available for each specific complaint. Acupressure and TNS are designed to act as simple and safe pain relieving techniques. Providing the instructions outlined are followed, they can be used without fear of adverse reaction or damage.

The third section describes a number of psychological techniques that can be used to help pain. These techniques will not in themselves act as pain-killers, but will help those suffering from pain to cope more effectively with their problems. A number of approaches are described, and these are prefaced by some introductory information which should help you to decide on the technique that you feel is most applicable to your personality. Again, those wishing to use the psychological techniques will need to read the introduction to the third section with some care so that they can decide on the most appropriate approach to their specific condition.

Acupressure, TNS and the relaxation techniques that are described can be used either for acute or for chronic pain. In some instances you may find that using a combination of a physical and psychological treatment will produce the best result. You must find the best approach to your pain; it is quite reasonable to consider the use of a combination of techniques in order to obtain the best pain relieving effects.

We have deliberately not covered the use of pain-killers, but have concentrated on the use of safe, simple and natural methods of providing pain relief. Our aim has been to suggest approaches to pain that mobilize the body's own natural healing powers from both the physical and psychological viewpoints. We hope that these measures will be effective in helping you, although it is important for you to realize that there is a wide range of conventional medications and procedures (such as injections or operations) which are important, often essential, treatments in the control and management of painful conditions. The use of such conventional management must always be considered in the light of your diagnosis and the cause of your pain. Therefore, in order to obtain the best method of pain management, please see your doctor before embarking on treatments outlined in this book. Your doctor will be able to make an accurate diagnosis of your pain and will therefore be able to tell you if other treatments are more appropriate for your particular condition.

GEORGE LEWITH & SANDRA HORN
Southampton, 1987

SECTION I

1. What is Pain?

Everyone knows what pain is from first-hand experience. Scraped shins, pin pricks, toothache, muscular spasm, back strain — all are almost universal phenomena. Some pains serve a useful purpose. They are urgent and unpleasant sensations, producing a strong need in us to make them stop. They are symptoms of disorder or disease. They may prompt us to take rapid evasive action, as in snatching a hand away from a hot iron; or perhaps to reduce our level of activity and to rest so as to aid recovery; or to seek help from a doctor, dentist, or analgesic medicine. These types of pain help us to adapt our behaviour so as to enhance our chances of survival. They tell us that damage to our body tissues is imminent, and we must do something *now* to prevent it. Pain is an unpleasant experience; it feels dangerous, and this helps to goad us into action. The onset of pain is frequently accompanied by activation of the sympathetic part of the nervous system. This produces effects such as raised blood-pressure, increased heart-rate and respiration, and so on, as part of the nervous system's alerting mechanism. Again, this prepares us for rapid action to deal with the cause of the pain.

The heightened emotional state accompanying pain helps to etch the experience into the memory, so that we learn to avoid the pain-producing situation in the future. A child may not learn to avoid pain by being told that something is hot and it will hurt, but if it touches the hot object once and *is* hurt, it is unlikely to do the same again.

This simple view of pain is adequate as far as it goes. Pain of the acute type is a symptom of damage to body tissue. However, this model is not able to explain a whole range of other types of pain. There are pains with no obvious injury or disease to account for them. There are pains which had a known cause originally, but which persist long after that cause has healed or gone. Pains can even come from tissue which is no longer there, as experienced by some people after amputation. There are 'trigger zones' which, when stimulated, can turn on pain in another area. Pain can be experienced in one place when the damage is elsewhere; this is so-called 'referred pain'. These observations demonstrate that there is no fixed relationship between injury and pain, and that pain can have no function. In such cases, pain must be regarded and treated as a problem in its own right.

Investigating pain

In the laboratory, clear relationships have been demonstrated between the feelings of a painful stimulus such as an electric shock or hard pressure on the skin, and its actual intensity. Not only the felt strength of the stimulus, but also its unpleasantness, can be related to the known physical measurements of the stimulus. However, in real life the story of pain is more complex and baffling. Things like memory, context and many personal, social and cultural factors intervene so as to modify the experience of pain dramatically. A football player receiving a kick on the shin as he is running for the ball at a crucial stage in the match might feel it as nothing much. An equivalent blow to an elderly person who falls could generate very much more pain.

We cannot measure pain directly. It can only be estimated from the subjective report of the sufferer. Even when scales are devised so that a score can be given for severity of pain, the number on the score has no absolute value. It only tells us how much that person feels they are suffering. Various attempts have been made to construct scales measuring pain. The visual analogue scale invites the scorer to estimate where the pain comes on a line representing intensity from 0 to 100 by making a mark on the line at the appropriate place.

No   0 |_____| 100   Worst possible
pain   pain

There are also descriptive scales:
'Ring the number most closely similar to the pain you are experiencing now.'
1. No pain   4. Severe pain
2. Mild pain   5. Excruciating pain
3. Moderate pain

Other scales relate pain to function, so that people can indicate how much the pain affects everyday activities such as walking:

Walking causes me no pain
Walking causes me some pain
Walking causes me severe pain
Walking is impossible because of pain

Yet other measures rely on observer reports, as when the incidence of, for example, grimacing, writhing, crying, or asking for medicine for pain, is recorded. These are the outward signs of distress, where the assumed cause is pain.

All these measures may be of some help in estimating pain; they can be useful in hospitals, for example, in trying to decide if a new drug or procedure or regime diminishes pain. However, as all rely on subjective and/or self-reporting experiences, they can only be rough guides at best, and are fraught with problems of interpretation.

Individual differences

Many things may influence the self-report or subjective experience of pain. Some people are by nature anxious and may tend to focus their anxieties on bodily health and be acutely affected by pain. Others may be very worried by pain if there is no convincing explanation for it, or if they fear it may have a sinister underlying cause, such as cancer, which has not been detected. In some, the pain may be a constant reminder of an unpleasant event such as an accident, so that it is associated in that person's mind with a tangle of negative emotions and unhappy memories, which serve to heighten the experience of pain. Yet others are, by nature, people who see life in very black and white terms; something is either there in its entirety or not there at all. All these people may describe and feel their pain as severe and incapacitating, or as causing 100 per cent distress. Conversely, fear, or a certain kind of temperament or upbringing, may lead people to underplay the impact of the pain and to be low scorers. While people are reporting their pain some will appear calm or even cheerful, some will look ill and drawn. It is all but impossible to make meaningful comparisons between all these people. Each one has a different personal style, and each one's pain is uniquely felt. At best, whether we use number scores or not, we 'guesstimate' pain in others. Looking at the differences between people is often a more fruitful line of study than trying to draw commonalities from numerical measures.

Other influences

Societies, cultures and families adopt attitudes to the expression of pain which will colour the individual's freedom to show or describe it — perhaps even to feel it. 'Big boys don't cry' — 'Stiff upper lip' and so on tell us what is and is not acceptable to others in our behaviour. We conform, or face scorn and disapproval. These are powerful influences on behaviour.

Prevailing circumstances also colour our behaviour. Studies on soldiers and civilians with post-operative pain showed that where the operation meant that the soldier would be taken out of the danger of active service and sent home, he showed less pain behaviour and needed fewer drugs than the civilian for whom the operation had no such positive outcome. Pain had different meaning for the two groups.

Fear may increase the subjective experience of pain, but extreme fear can block out pain altogether. There are reports of people wounded in battle and feeling no pain while they were fighting for their lives. Only when they were out of danger did they feel pain from their wounds. There is also an account from an explorer being mauled by a lion; he was so terrified that he felt completely numb while the lion was tearing at his flesh. Emotions can change the perception of pain.

The anticipation of pain can also cause it to be felt as worse. Children subjected to a painful procedure, such as dressing-changes on burnt skin, begin to show all the distress associated with pain before the procedure begins, as time goes on, because they anticipate the pain. In such cases they do not adapt; each new episode begins in anxious anticipation and seems to cause more pain.

Our experience of pain, then, is very individual. It is determined by a combination of the sort of person we are, our upbringing, our state at the onset of pain, the antecedent and surrounding events, and our understanding of the consequences of it. Pain is universally known and yet a uniquely personal experience. It can be a simple and well-understood signal of tissue damage, or a mysterious phenomenon with no demonstrable organic cause. When it is the latter, and has also become chronic or recurrent, it can be a potent source of ongoing stress to the sufferer, and may have devastating long-term effects.

Long-term effects of chronic pain

In spite of individual differences in response to pain in the short or medium term, chronic pain tends to produce a recognized behaviour pattern in many people. Pain is a physical and psychological stressor. Like other kinds of stress-generating events, it tends to keep the sufferer in an almost constant state of alertness or arousal, as a response to the feeling of threat it brings with it. This state is often accompanied by increased muscle tension, and by feelings of anxiety or irritability. Increased muscle tension may be associated with the site of the pain; it is often an instinctive response to pain, as if to assist the healing process by keeping the injured part still and not subjecting it to further damage by moving it. However, in chronic pain this response will serve only to add to the pain, as muscles around the site become stiff and tense. Nevertheless, it is a hard habit to break.

The constant stress caused by chronic pain may ultimately lead to depression, as do many other sources of anxiety and distress which fail to remit. Disturbances of sleep, appetite and energy levels are common in depression, and irritability may be accompanied by increasing apathy, so that even the short spurts of energy provided by an outburst of irritability cannot be used purposefully.

Another effect of chronic pain, allied to apathy but not necessarily the same, is a gradual diminution of activity. This often begins with abandoning actions which cause an increase in pain, such as lifting shopping bags or walking long distances. The problem is that the reduction in activity usually fails to stop there. The anxiety about causing extra pain tends to spread to similar pieces of behaviour, so that someone who, perhaps wisely, abandoned lifting heavy shopping bags, may end by abandoning lifting pots and pans, and so relinquish cooking and then other activities as well. Many people also find that rest relieves pain and, as they do less, they rest more. Over a number of months, some pain sufferers find that they are spending much of the day in bed or on the sofa, while their daily activities have been reduced to very little indeed. Such strategies rarely control pain effectively, however. Most of these pain sufferers will be in as much pain as ever, but they fear to do more because they might make the pain worse. They are caught in a trap.

Another aspect of chronic pain and its effect on behaviour is the tendency for there to be an ever-increasing reliance on pain-killing drugs, most of which soon lose their effectiveness. The trap is the same as the trap of doing little and resting much; it does not significantly help the pain, but the fear that stopping will make it worse, maintains the behaviour. The long-term use of strong pain-killers is undesirable in many cases of chronic pain, and they tend to have unhelpful side-effects such as constipation and clouding of consciousness. Some are also habit-forming, and will make the sufferer feel ill for a while if he or she tries to cut them down too rapidly. It is easier to go on taking them.

This picture of the chronic pain sufferer is a sad one. Feeling low, doing little, absorbed in the pain, swallowing tablets. When pain dominates all of life to this extent, it is worth considering alternative ways of coping with it. Some people come to these ways naturally; they refuse to give in and they find ways round pain-producing activities. Not everyone is so lucky. In this book, a number of pain management strategies are described, which may help some sufferers to find a better way of coping. THEY SHOULD NOT BE TRIED WITHOUT DISCUSSION WITH A MEDICAL ADVISER, AS THE PAIN MAY BE ARISING FROM ACTIVE TISSUE DAMAGE REQUIRING MEDICAL OR SURGICAL INTERVENTION. THEY ARE INTENDED FOR USE WITH PAIN WHERE NO INTERVENTION OF THAT TYPE IS APPROPRIATE — which means that they will have been properly diagnosed, or at least that treatable organic pathology will have been ruled out as a cause. No one should try to deal with a pain they have not discussed with their medical adviser.

The methods of pain control used in the book are of two types; physical and psychological. The physical methods are acupressure, in which pressure is applied to certain of the acupuncture points described in traditional Chinese medicine to block pain; and transcutaneous electrical nerve stimulation (TNS), in which a mild electrical current applied across the skin can inhibit the transmission of pain sensation through the nervous system. The psychological methods are relaxation, meditation, autogenic hypnosis and visual imagery, all of which use our natural abilities to attain a degree of control over some bodily functions, including those pertaining to the perception of pain. All the techniques are described in sufficient detail to allow them to be used by pain sufferers who wish to take effective control of their pain without recourse to excessive drug-taking, and who have established with their medical practitioner that it is safe for them to do so.

Understanding the cause of your pain

All pain arises in the first instance because the brain interprets a changed state somewhere in the body's cells as damaging or potentially damaging. Usually a certain amount of change has already happened, and the brain signals 'pain' to prevent it getting worse. The signal 'pain' is urgent and unpleasant, and goads us into rapid action to change things. So far, so good. However, we know that many ongoing pains no longer fit this model. Why do we go on feeling pain if no further damage is occurring? Why does a scar from an operation heal up painlessly, and then begin to hurt later, when the surgeon says that the operation was entirely successful and that the scar is a 'good' one? Why do we feel pain from an amputated ('phantom') limb? Why does shingles sometimes go on hurting for months, or even in some unfortunate cases years, after the rash has disappeared? How can a bad back go on and on hurting when all the investigations and X-rays are normal?

These are the sort of questions which tend to preoccupy people with long-term pain, and they need answers, or they can become a source of fretful worrying, which is far from helpful.

Signalling pain

All over the body hundreds of thousands of sensory nerve-endings are regularly receiving and transmitting information to the brain. Those nerve-endings which transmit signals about tissue damage are small diameter nerve fibres which fire all the time. When a painful stimulus occurs, they increase their rate of firing. They are presumably sending signals to the brain all the time, which say that everything is normal. When something 'not normal' like a cut or an area of inflammation occurs, they signal 'change from normal' and the brain may interpret that as pain. The 'change' signal must be transmitted, received, *and* interpreted by the brain for the pain to be felt and, as we have seen, many factors can influence that perception.

There is evidence from research which suggests that sometimes the pathways involved in transmitting noxious (painful) stimuli show long-lasting changes as a result of being triggered. A stimulus resulting in a burst of firing in those nerves can also cause changes in other nerve-endings in adjacent tissues. Then, nerves which had been transmitting 'touch' begin signalling 'pain'. This means that the input into the nervous system from that area is changed in a significant way, and it could be one reason why pain goes on being felt, even after the original stimulus has gone. It is not that damage is still being done, but that the original stimulus has caused a change in the nervous system with long-term results.

There are also long-term effects when a nerve has been cut, or damaged by stretching or crushing, so that fibres within the nerve become disconnected. When this happens, the nerve fibres below the cut degenerate. Those above, which are still connected to their cell bodies, will grow down into the damaged area but may not reach their proper target tissue. The scrambled messages generated by this new distribution of the nerve fibres may predispose the brain to interpret them as pain, perhaps because the signals are saying 'different from normal' (i.e. potential damage).

When severed nerves cannot grow back to their targets, as in amputation, they often form tangled bunches (neuromas) on the cut ends, which fire spontaneously and which may result in the sensation of continuous pain.

In all these ways the input to the central nervous system is changed in a way which generates the experience of pain in the absence of further injury. The initial noxious stimulus — stretching, pinching, crushing, cutting, irritating — has become irrelevant, but the pain remains to be dealt with. Sometimes pain can be successfully abolished by bombarding the nerve-endings with weak electrical stimuli (Transcutaneous Electrical Nerve Stimulation) which seem to be received by the brain at the expense of the pain stimuli. This well-established principle, the gate control theory of pain, will be explained and expanded in Chapter 2. Input to the central nervous system can also be influenced in a similar way by the use of acupressure and related techniques.

Central factors

Just as certain features of the input from nerve-endings can be changed to block the experience of pain, factors operating centrally (that is, on the brain) can be changed too. Pain can be enhanced by anxiety or stress, and diminished by relaxation. In response to pain, the brain can stimulate the release of the body's natural pain-killers or endorphins. It may be that techniques like acupuncture, relaxation, meditation and hypnosis also help to produce endorphin release. When these techniques are applied successfully, they produce not only pain relief, but a sense of well-being in keeping with the morphine-like action of the body's own natural pain-killers. In using these techniques, we may be tapping into a natural mechanism in a systematic way.

The other important aspect of central factors in pain, already mentioned previously, is attention. Pain naturally focuses the attention on itself because it feels dangerous. Switching the attention away diminishes the pain and can sometimes abolish it altogether. Again, this is the conscious and systematic use of a natural attribute. When pain is present but has no function and no meaning, it is like a rogue signal or a scrambled message which keeps on getting into a communication system. Taking strong drugs to damp down the signal may affect the whole system but still fail to abolish the rogue signal. Natural methods use blocking techniques specifically directed to the malfunctioning system. They do no harm to the overall functioning of the nervous system, and moreover their actions can be understood by those who want to use them, as has been shown.

Understanding pain, and understanding pain-control mechanisms, can only be to the good of the pain sufferer seeking self-help. Understanding is a necessary part of being in control. It also helps to allay the fear that pain *must* mean that something sinister is going on. We now know that damage or disturbance to certain peripheral nerves can generate pain over long periods of time, and that pain can sometimes etch a kind of memory of itself into the central nervous system, which can also maintain pain after the original cause has gone. These are pains without function.

In addition to those types of pain, there are others with an organic cause of a relatively minor type. These do not suggest that anything sinister or progressive is going on. Headache (when it is not a symptom of disease) is a good example. The pain might be caused by relatively small changes in pressure or tension, in blood vessels or muscles. These pains can be extremely worrying until they are properly diagnosed and explained. The worry makes the pain worse. Understanding what is going on can sometimes be enough in itself to make the pain bearable and manageable. It is always important to have your pain diagnosed and explained for these reasons. Then, when you know that your pain is functionless or at least *not* a symptom of a disease or disorder which itself needs attention, you will be in a position to consider self-help techniques such as those described here.

SECTION II

2. An Introduction to Acupuncture and Transcutaneous Nerve Stimulation

The development of Chinese medicine

Acupuncture, or needle puncture, is a European term invented by Willem Ten Rhyne, a Dutch physician who visited Nagasaki in Japan, in the early part of the seventeenth century. The Chinese describe acupuncture by the character 'Chen', which literally means, 'to prick with a needle'. Acupuncture and the closely related technique of acupressure have a recorded history of about 2,000 years, but some authorities claim that they have been practised in China for much longer. The Chinese believe that stone knives or sharp-edged tools were used some 4,000 years ago to puncture and drain abscesses; these instruments were called 'Bian' stones. The character 'Bian' means the use of a sharp-edged stone to treat disease. The modern Chinese character 'Bi' describes a disease of pain and is almost certainly derived from the use of 'Bian' stones for the treatment of painful complaints. Pressing over these points, or acupressure, probably has a very similar history.

The origin of Chinese medicine is a complex story, and acupuncture/acupressure represents only one facet of the development of this system. The first recorded attempt at treating disease dates back to about 1500 BC; tortoise shells with inscriptions dating from that time were thought to have been used in the art of healing. The philosophical basis for much of very early Chinese medicine seems to have been to seek harmony between the living and their dead ancestors, and the good and evil spirits that inhabited the earth.

The first known acupuncture text is the *Nei Ching Su Wen*. This book is also known by a variety of alternative titles such as the *Yellow Emperor's Classic of Internal Medicine*, or the *Canon of Medicine*. The initial section of the *Nei Ching Su Wen* involves a discussion between the Yellow Emperor, Huang Ti, and his

Minister, Ch'i Pai, which lays down the framework of traditional Chinese medical thought. The authorship of the *Nei Ching Su Wen* is attributed to Huang Ti, but there is some doubt as to whether he actually existed and a great deal more uncertainty as to who wrote the book. It was probably written by a variety of people and seems to date from the Warring States period (475-221 BC).

The Western doctor observes the facts before him and uses the current scientific theories to explain them. Chinese medicine is based on a much wider world view, but one that is more difficult to justify and almost impossible to test. These ideas are woven into a complete system based on a philosophy different from that of Western medicine; for instance, the concept of yin and yang and the number 5 are two of the more important factors in much of traditional Chinese scientific thought.

The Warring States period is a particularly interesting time in Chinese history and has exerted a great deal of influence on Chinese thought. Two main philosophical ideologies emerged during this time, Taoism and Confucianism. Confucianism defined the social status of prince and pauper within Chinese society and elected the Emperor a god. It resulted in a basically feudal and totalitarian system of government that exists today in an adapted form. Taoism represented quite a different approach; the Tao literally means the 'way' and the philosophy of Taoism is a method of maintaining harmony between man and his world, and between this world and beyond. The Taoist concept of health is to attempt to attain perfect harmony between the opposing forces of the natural world — between yin and yang — the belief being that the only way to be healthy is to adjust to these natural forces and become part of their rhythm. Furthermore, such forces are completely dependent on each other: earth is dependent on rain and rain is dependent on heaven, which in turn cannot exist without earth. The concept of a unified force governing natural events is central to much of Chinese scientific thought.

At first glance these concepts seem to be an irrelevant sideline to the development of a system of medicine. In essence the ideal of health is perfect harmony between the forces of yin and yang. However, this state is rarely attained and most of us exist in a state of variable health: one day we feel well and the next day less well. All of us are in a state of change, but it is only when this change causes irreversible disharmony that it results in established disease.

Pain is one of the symptoms of the disharmony described by traditional Chinese medicine, and techniques based on puncturing or pressing acupuncture points are designed to relieve pain by (in traditional Chinese terms) restoring harmonious relationships in the body.

Acupuncture in the West
It is probable that acupuncture has been used in the West since the seventeenth century, but its first recorded use was by Dr Berlioz at the Paris Medical School in 1810. He treated a young woman suffering from abdominal pain, and although the Paris Medical School described this as a reckless form of treatment, Dr Berlioz continued to use acupuncture and claimed great success with it.

Acupuncture and acupressure are not new to England. The first known British acupuncturist was John Churchill, who, in 1821, published a series of results on the treatment of rheumatism with acupuncture. In 1823 acupuncture was mentioned in the first issue of the *Lancet*, and in 1824 Dr Elliotson, a physician at St Thomas's Hospital, London, began to use this method of treatment. In 1827 he published a paper describing the treatment of forty-two cases of rheumatism by acupuncture and concluded that this was an effective approach to such problems.

Electro-acupuncture and transcutaneous nerve stimulation (TNS)
During the 1950s the Chinese began to produce electrical stimulators that allowed a small amount of pulsed electrical current to pass between sets of paired acupuncture needles. These were initially used to replace the prolonged manual stimulation of acupuncture needles during acupuncture anaesthesia.

The use and effects of such electrical stimulators has been examined in great detail by many medical researchers. We now know that acupuncture, acupressure and a variety of electrical stimulation techniques will produce pain relief by activating particular nerve pathways and chemicals within the body. This led people to ask whether needles were really necessary; perhaps the electrical current would be just as effective if passed through small electro-conductive pads directly in contact with the skin? During the late 1960s and early 1970s small portable battery operated machines called transcutaneous nerve stimulators (TNS) were developed.

The machine itself is a portable battery-operated stimulator that generates small-amplitude, pulsed square waves. These electrical transmissions travel via small wires to electrodes placed directly on the skin, often on or around the painful site. TNS machines and their action are described in greater detail in Chapter 5.

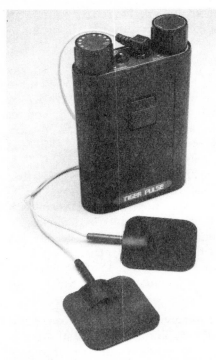

Figure 1. An RDG Tiger Pulse TNS machine produced by RDG Electro-Medical Equipment (429 Brighton Road, Croydon, Surrey, CR2 6UD). The cost of the basic unit, including leads and reusable pads, is £56.90 (exclusive of VAT).

Figure 2. The Neen Microtens produced by Neen Pain Products (Barn Lodge, Gooseberry Hill, Swanton Morley, Dereham, Norfolk, NR20 4NR). The cost of the basic unit, including leads and reusable pads, is £57.90 (exclusive of VAT).

Prices quoted as of April 1986.

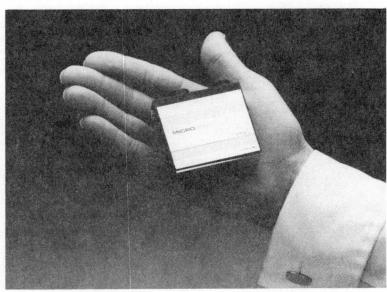

Two different but similar systems

TNS and acupressure are therefore essentially similar techniques in that they both use the same basic information which has its roots in acupuncture. They represent two slightly different ways of stimulating the body to mobilize its own natural defences against many diseases, particularly pain.

Western doctors have become fascinated by acupuncture over the last ten to fifteen years. This was largely generated by President Nixon's renewed political interest in all things Chinese, including acupuncture anaesthesia. New theories on the perception and transmission of pain also played their part; some of these new ideas were thought to explain how acupuncture and acupressure might actually work.

Painful points

The development of acupuncture points on the body demonstrates an interesting story of rediscovery. Over the last fifty years many Western physicians have noted independently that pressing, stimulating or injecting various points on or just under the skin

Figure 3. The Pulsar produced by Spembly Medical Ltd (Newbury Road, Andover, Hants, SP10 4DR). The cost of the basic unit, including leads and reusable pads, is £58.00 (exclusive of VAT).

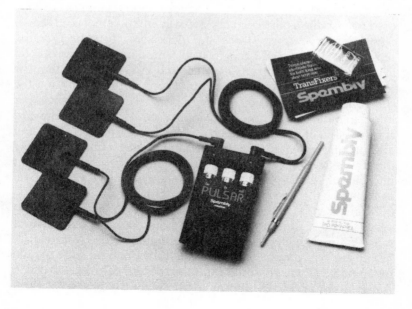

can help to relieve pain, particularly pain caused by injury to the muscles, bones and joints. These points are not necessarily at the site of pain, but often over distant areas. For instance, arthritis of the neck frequently presents with pain over the shoulder and shoulder blade. On a close examination it is often possible to define the origin of the pain and demonstrate that the neck is the cause of the problem. However, acupressure or stimulation of the painful points around the shoulder blade often relieves the pain and frees neck movement. These 'trigger points' correlate very closely with acupuncture points. There have been a number of attempts to understand the existence of trigger points but, as yet, no clear explanation of this phenomenon. It is interesting to note that the Chinese realized this fact some 2,500 years ago and the *Ling Shu* (an ancient Chinese text) summarizes this approach when it says: 'In pain puncture the tender point.' We know that treating these special areas (or tender trigger points) is particularly useful in pain.

The effects on pain pathways and pain transmission
But how do acupuncture and TNS actually work? In 1965 two doctors, Melzack and Wall, proposed the gate control theory of pain. This stated that pain was transmitted from the periphery (for instance a burnt finger) to the spinal cord via small diameter nerve fibres. These fibres terminated in the spinal cord, in a structure called the substantia gelatinosa. The substantia gelatinosa is a term used to describe a particular site actually in the spinal cord. Large diameter nerve fibres from the periphery, usually carrying sensations such as light touch, also terminate in the substantia gelatinosa. It seemed from Melzack and Wall's research that the transmission of pain from the spinal cord to the brain (and the subsequent perception of pain) could be altered by large fibre input into the spinal cord. This type of input seemed to stop the onward transmission of pain and thereby, 'close the gate to pain'. TNS and acupuncture appear to stimulate the large diameter fibres selectively thereby decreasing the painful excitation caused by small-fibre input into the substantia gelatinosa. This alters our perception of pain as it blocks the onward transmission of painful stimuli.

More recently, in the mid 1970s, naturally occurring chemicals very similar to opium were isolated from the nervous system of many animals including humans. Opium and its close relative heroin are very powerful pain-killers. If their natural release could be stimulated then we would expect significant pain relief to occur. Acupressure and TNS appear to stimulate the release of these natural opioids (usually called endorphins and enkephalins) and can, through this mechanism, modify and relieve pain. The effects of this natural increase in 'home made' pain-killers can be largely reversed by drugs that antagonize the effect of heroin and opium in the body.

These two mechanisms provide us with a very clear understanding of how these simple techniques can actually alleviate pain in a very consistent manner. In fact it might be said that we know more about how acupuncture works than we do about the mechanisms behind such commonly used drugs as aspirin!

Traditional Chinese medicine

The Chinese system of medicine suggests that health is achieved and disease prevented by maintaining the body in a balanced state. The Chinese believe that two opposing forces exist in the natural world, yin (water, tranquillity and femininity) and yang (fire, activity and masculinity). Vital energy or *qi* circulates through the body and keeps these forces in balance. A normal fluctuating balance of yin and yang should exist in the healthy individual, which is why we feel better on some days than others!

Traditional Chinese medicine also contains a myriad of laws that govern the selection of acupuncture points and describe in exact detail the function of a whole variety of organs. In fact some of the organ functions described by the ancient Chinese predate by many hundreds of years their 'discovery' in the West. For instance, the Chinese discovered the double circulation of blood long before Western medicine realized that it existed.

We shall be discussing the fourteen main acupuncture channels as these provide a very useful basis upon which to decide the best treatment for a particular condition. We do not intend to discuss the detailed body of information that underpins much of traditional Chinese medical thought. However, it is important to realize that this knowledge provides us with the information used in the disease section as it helps considerably with point selection. Those readers who are interested in studying traditional Chinese medicine further should read G.T. and N.R. Lewith, *Modern Chinese Acupuncture* (Thorsons, 1984). Porkert M. *The Theoretical Foundations of Chinese Medicine*, (MIT Press, 1978) provides a very detailed discussion of traditional Chinese philosophy and this book will be of interest to the specialist.

The comparative value of acupressure and TNS

Pain should be treated initially as a symptom and not as a diagnosis in itself. Therefore if you or any of your friends are suffering from pain it is vital that you know the cause of the pain before beginning to treat it. If the pain is the result of a cancer or a burst appendix then it may be quite inappropriate to use acupressure or TNS to relieve the pain without being fully aware of the diagnosis and all the other treatments available.

Several questions often occur to patients who suffer pain, the most important one being; will this treatment work for me? No treatment is a guaranteed cure for any chronic pain. Acupressure and TNS will probably provide some benefit for two thirds to three quarters of patients suffering from chronic pain as a consequence of conditions such as acute injury or arthritis. In effect this means that these simple techniques are always worth trying providing you know what has caused the pain and that therefore you are not actively masking symptoms in a potentially dangerous situation. We have all read, with growing frequency and concern, about the adverse reactions which can result from conventional medication (particularly for conditions such as arthritis). Techniques such as acupressure and TNS are really very safe.

One technique isn't really better than another. Patients who respond to TNS are likely to respond to acupressure and vice versa. In a sense acupressure is a much simpler and cheaper technique to practise as there is no necessity to purchase a machine. However, acupressure often requires the help of a friend or a relative should the painful area be over the lower back or in the middle of the spine. TNS can be handled by the patient alone and used throughout a busy working day where it might be inconvenient or impossible to use acupressure over prolonged periods. We will therefore describe both techniques so you can decide on the most appropriate approach to your problem. We would advise the use of simple acupressure initially, and if this fails to produce a consistent response then your general practitioner, physiotherapist or any other attending doctor should be consulted about the value of purchasing a TNS machine.

3. Acupuncture Points and Channels

The evolution of acupuncture points and channels
Acupuncture points are undoubtedly the end product of millions of detailed observations and, as they were developed, so each of them was given a Chinese name which implied its functional and clinical importance. There is an instinctive urge to cause more pain over a painful area; the image of a person with toothache pressing on the painful tooth is a frequent cartoonist's joke. As has already been suggested, common painful diseases consistently cause painful points to emerge in well-defined locations on the body. When such a point is stimulated the pain can be alleviated, hence the idea of a point for treating pain. From this simple beginning it is easy to see how a system of acupuncture points evolved for the management of painful conditions.

Acupuncture points were subsequently grouped into a system of channels which run over the body. The channels are said to conduct the flow of vital energy or qi through the body. Furthermore, each channel or group of acupuncture points was designated with the name of an organ. Although we shall not be using many of the assumptions made by the traditional Chinese about the treatment of internal disease, we shall for the sake of continuity and completeness continue to name the channels after their designated organ. In spite of the fact that the existence of channels has never been scientifically proven, they do provide a very useful and practical framework for selecting acupuncture points in the treatment of pain as well as many other conditions.

The principles of therapy
The Chinese think of pain as a symptom caused by a disruption or 'blockage' to the free flow of vital energy or qi through the channels. It is almost as if the symptom pain has resulted from

the physical disruption of the channels and their internal connections. They believe that the flow of qi can be normalized (and the pain subsequently resolved) by one of two main methods:

1. The treatment of *local tender* points on or around the channel traversing the site of injury.
2. The treatment of local points over the painful area and the use of *distal points* on the channel or channels running over the pain. Distal points have no logical rhyme or reason behind them. They are at points near the hand or the foot, on channels that run over the painful areas. They are, however, of enormous practical value in the management of painful conditions and their use should be considered each time you treat your pain.

This means that if someone is suffering from shoulder pain then points around the shoulder can be used as well as distal points on the large intestine channel, running over the shoulder. (See *Figure 4*.)

Painful points do not always occur on the channels. These 'ouch' or 'Ah Shi' points should always be treated in painful conditions. Ah Shi is simply the Chinese term to describe a particularly painful, small, area on the body. Ideally the point that is most tender should be localized and treated first. There may be one central tender point, which when treated results in relief over the whole painful area. However, more frequently a number of such tender or Ah Shi points will require therapy. Some of these points will be found on the channels while others may be closely related to the channels and will simply be noted as tender points.

The direction of the flow of qi up and down the channels is also important. When using acupressure the points chosen should be, as far as possible, massaged in the same direction as the flow of qi. The direction of the flow of qi will be clearly marked in the diagrams on pages 33 to 48 which demonstrate the course of each of the fourteen main channels. When using TNS this flow of qi appears to be less important than placing the negative (black) electrode on the site of greatest pain or injury. Any distal points should have a positive or red electrode placed upon them. Therefore when using acupressure, massage in the direction that the channel is said to be 'flowing', and when using TNS, stimulate the site of injury or greatest pain with a small negative current.

General points
In the chapter describing treatment for each particular condition, we also define a third group of points: general points. These points

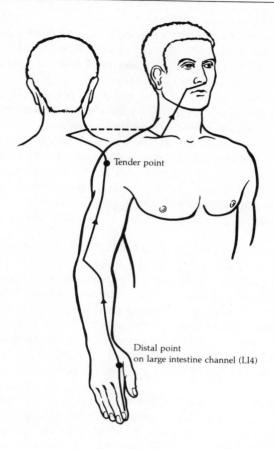

Figure 4. This is the large intestine channel with the tender point on the shoulder marked. In order to treat using either acupressure or TNS, the tender point should be treated along with the appropriate distal point (LI4).

are firmly rooted in traditional Chinese medicine and are designed to 'balance' the body so that the internal aspect of any illness may be treated. If you have pain for a prolonged period of time then this almost invariably results in other symptoms such as depression (because of the pain), indigestion (because of the pain-killers) or sometimes constipation (also because of the pain-killers taken). Many other symptoms may also be present. The general points are designed to treat the internal aspects of chronic conditions and are particularly important in illnesses such as migraine headaches.

The channels: how to use them

There are fourteen main channels, eight of which are used largely to treat internal diseases and six of which are used in painful conditions. All the channels are represented *bilaterally* on the body except for the Ren and Du channels which are unilateral. In pain you should start by treating local and distal points on the painful side and if necessary then treat your chosen points bilaterally. General points should always be treated bilaterally from the outset.

The points needed for each particular disease are defined accurately in the individual sections in Chapter 6. The six channels used most frequently for the treatment of pain all have distal points, the other channels do not. These distal points form the basic grammar of acupuncture and are particularly effective, especially if the treatment of local points alone fails to produce adequate results.

The diagrams that follow illustrate each of the fourteen channels giving the direction of flow of qi (for use in acupressure) and the relevant distal points (for use in acupressure and TNS). Try to remember the distribution of the channels over the body. One or more distal points may be used to treat pain, depending on the distribution of the pain over the body. For instance a shoulder pain may travel over the small intestine, large intestine and sanjiao channels. Those using acupressure may need to massage large intestine 4, sanjiao 5 and small intestine 3 in order to get an adequate result.

The point numbers referred to throughout this text simply define the point and replace the naming systems originally used by traditional acupuncturists. The point numbering system used is the Chinese system, for those who may wish to refer to other acupuncture or acupressure texts.

The total of fourteen channels is made up of six channels running from the head to the arm represented on both sides of the body, six channels running from the head to the legs represented on both sides of the body and two 'central' channels. Three channels in the arm are used for the treatment of pain (small intestine, large intestine and sanjiao) and three channels in the arm are used, largely, for the treatment of internal disease (heart, lung and pericardium). Three channels in the leg are used for the treatment of pain (urinary bladder, gall-bladder and stomach) and three channels are used largely for the treatment of internal disease (spleen, kidney and liver). The Ren and Du channels are central and are extra channels usually used for the treatment of internal diseases.

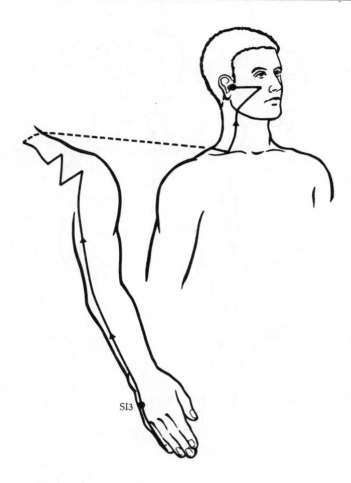

Figure 5 The small intestine channel

1. *The small intestine channel* (*Figure 5*)
(The small intestine channel is abbreviated to SI)
The distribution of the small intestine channel starts at the root of the little finger nail and travels up the back of the arm over the shoulder blade ending just in front of the ear.

The only important distal point on the small intestine channel is SI3 — this is marked.

The direction of the flow of qi in the channel is marked with an arrow.

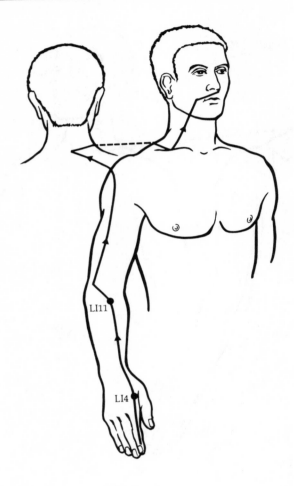

Figure 6　The large intestine channel

2. *The large intestine channel* (*Figure 6*)
(The large intestine channel is abbreviated to LI)
The distribution of the large intestine channel starts at the nail of
the first finger and passes up the front of the arm over the shoulder
to the face, ending at the side of the nostril.

The distal points on the channel are LI4 and LI11 — these are
marked. The direction of the flow of qi in the channel is marked
with an arrow.

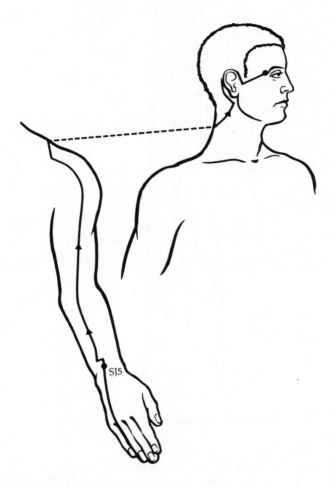

Figure 7 The sanjiao channel

3. *The sanjiao channel* (*Figure 7*)
(The sanjiao channel is abbreviated to SJ)
The distribution of the sanjiao channel begins at the tip of the ring finger and runs up the middle of the back of the arm, over the tip of the shoulder to the ear and then to the outside of the eyebrow.

The distal point on the channel is SJ5 — this is marked.

The direction of the flow of qi in the channel is marked with an arrow.

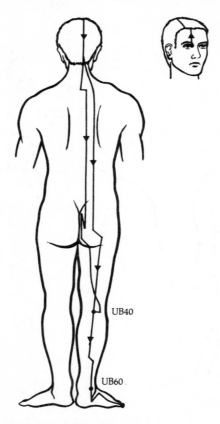

Figure 8   The urinary bladder channel

4. *The urinary bladder channel (Figure 8)*
(The urinary bladder channel is abbreviated to UB)
The distribution of the urinary bladder channel starts on the inside
of the eye, passes over the top of the head and then splits into two
over the middle of the back. It then passes down the spine and
leg as two channels, rejoining at the back of the knee, running
down the middle of the lower leg and the side of the foot, ending
finally on the outside of the little toe.

The distal points on the channel are UB40 for pain experienced
in the low back and UB60 for pain experienced in the middle or
upper back.

The direction of the flow of qi in the channel is marked with
an arrow.

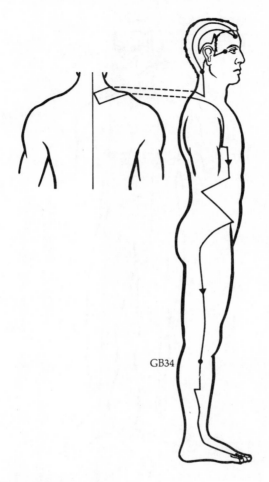

Figure 9   The gall-bladder channel

5. *The gall-bladder channel (Figure 9)*
(The gall-bladder channel is abbreviated to GB)
The distribution of the gall-bladder channel starts at the side of
the eye and runs over the side of the head, passing backwards and
forwards over the head. It then runs down over the shoulder,
abdomen and leg, ending on the side of the fourth toe.

The distal point on the channel is GB34 — this is marked.

The direction of the flow of qi in the channel is marked with
an arrow.

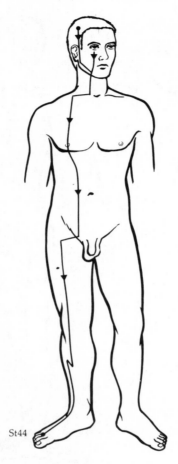

St44

Figure 10   The stomach channel

6. *The stomach channel (Figure 10)*
(The stomach channel is abbreviated to St)
The distribution of the stomach channel starts just below the eye, and then does a 'U' bend over the face passing down through the throat, over the abdomen down through the front of the thigh and into the foot; it passes between the second and third toes and ends at the root of the second toe nail.

The distal point on the channel is St44 — this is marked.

The direction of the flow of qi in the channel is marked with an arrow.

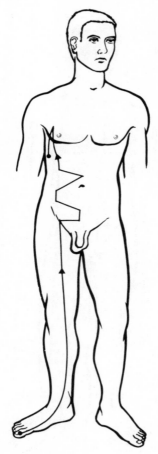

Figure 11 The spleen channel

7. *The spleen channel (Figure 11)*
(The spleen channel is abbreviated to Sp)
The distribution of the spleen channel starts on the big toe, then travels up the inside of the leg and thigh, over the genitalia, abdomen and thorax. After coming up to the chest, it ends in a line directly below the armpit.

There is no distal point as this is a channel for the treatment of internal diseases.

The direction of the flow of qi in the channel is marked with an arrow.

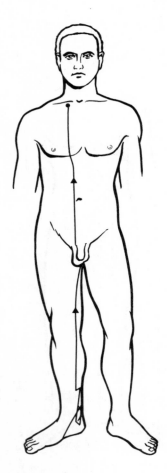

Figure 12   The kidney channel

8. *The kidney channel (Figure 12)*
(The kidney channel is abbreviated to K)
The distribution of the kidney channel starts on the sole of the foot, travels up the inner part of the leg and over the abdomen, ending at the top of the ribs.

There is no distal point as this is a channel for the treatment of internal diseases.

The direction of the flow of qi in the channel is marked with an arrow.

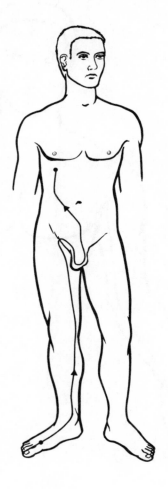

Figure 13   The liver channel

9. *The liver channel* (*Figure 13*)
(The liver channel is abbreviated to Liv)
The distribution of the liver channel starts on the big toe, running up the inner leg, over the abdomen to end just below the fourth rib.

There is no distal point as this is a channel for the treatment of internal diseases.

The direction of the flow of qi in the channel is marked with an arrow.

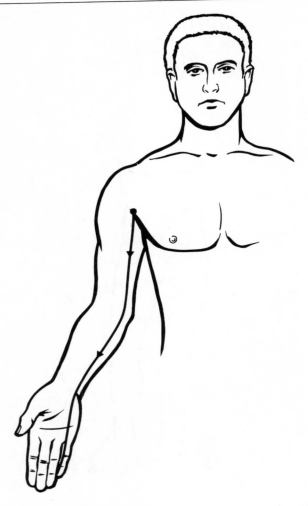

Figure 14 The heart channel

10. *The heart channel (Figure 14)*
(The heart channel is abbreviated to H)
The distribution of the heart channel starts in the armpit and runs down the front of the arm ending at the little fingernail.

There is no distal point as this is a channel for the treatment of internal diseases.

The direction of the flow of qi in the channel is marked with an arrow.

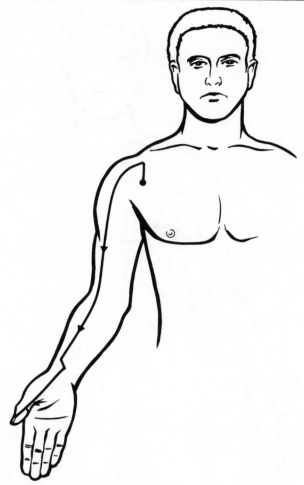

Figure 15   The lung channel

11. *The lung channel (Figure 15)*
(The lung channel is abbreviated to Lu)
The distribution of the lung channel starts on the front chest wall
between the first and second rib. It then passes down the front aspect
of the arm to the middle of the thumb.

There is no distal point as this is a channel for the treatment
of internal diseases.

The direction of the flow of qi in the channel is marked with
an arrow.

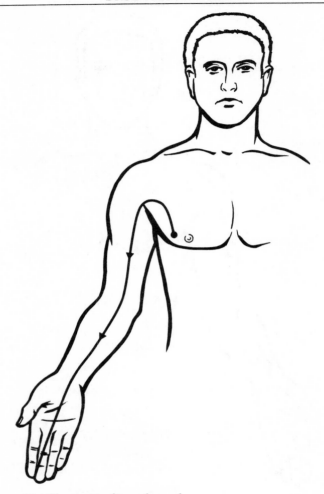

Figure 16 The pericardium channel

12. *The pericardium channel (Figure 16)*
(The pericardium channel is abbreviated to P)
The distribution of the pericardium channel starts on the thorax, just beside the nipple. It runs down the middle of the arm ending at the nail of the middle finger.

There is no distal point as this is a channel for the treatment of internal diseases.

The direction of the flow of qi in the channel is marked with an arrow.

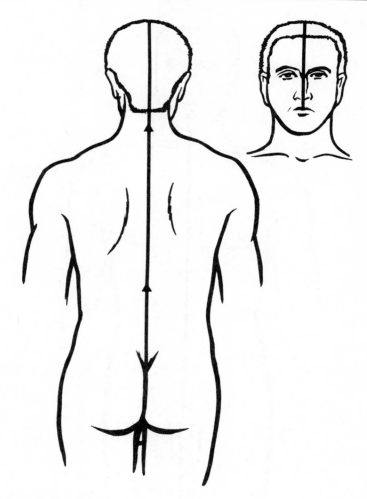

Figure 17 Du channel

13. *Du channel (Figure 17)*

This runs from the genitals to the upper lip, over the middle of the back, top of the head and into the upper lip. In some acupuncture texts it is called the governor vessel. There is only one Du channel on the body.

There is no distal point on this channel.

The direction of the flow of qi in the channel is marked with an arrow.

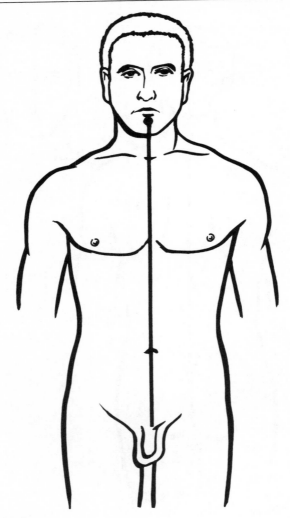

Figure 18   Ren channel

14. *Ren channel (Figure 18)*
This run from the genitals up over the abdomen and throat to the lower lip. In some acupuncture texts the Ren channel is called the conception channel. There is only one Ren channel on the body.

There is no distal point on this channel.

The direction of the flow of qi in the channel is marked with an arrow.

4. The Technique of Acupressure

Acupressure

We have already discussed some of the historical scientific background to acupuncture and acupressure. Probably the most important fact to remember in the treatment of any painful condition is: PAIN IS A SYMPTOM, AND CLEAR DIAGNOSIS AS TO ITS CAUSE IS ESSENTIAL. IF YOU DO NOT KNOW WHAT IS CAUSING YOUR PAIN THEN SEEK THE OPINION OF A QUALIFIED DOCTOR BEFORE YOU START TREATING YOURSELF. REMEMBER THAT PAIN IS OFTEN A WARNING SIGN GIVEN BY THE BODY, SO IT MUST BE HEEDED.

In Chapter 6, which deals with specific painful conditions, the exact points which can be used to treat specific painful problems are localized clearly on the diagrams provided. A short verbal description of the point location is also provided in the text.

Remember that in pain it is very important to localize the most painful point as carefully as you can and treat this point. On some occasions you will find that the painful point is not described on the diagrams provided. Most of the time pain originating from a specific joint or muscle follows a fairly standard distribution, but occasionally the distribution of pain from a painful knee or hip may be slightly unusual.

When practising acupressure it is essential to find the points as correctly as possible. The more accurately you massage the point the greater its effect. When localizing a point the following guidelines should be followed:

1. EXAMINE the painful area carefully in an effort to localize the most tender point as clearly as possible. If you can't get to the painful area (for instance, in the mid-back) then you may need to seek the help of a friend or relative as this will

make it much simpler for you to find the points on your own body.

2. VISUAL: Look carefully at the illustrations provided in order to localize the point or points on your own body.
3. READ the descriptions of the points carefully, as this will act as a useful adjunct to the diagrams provided.
4. SENSITIVITY over the acupuncture points will be greater than that of surrounding tissue.

As we have mentioned, you may well need help to find some of the points on the back. In order to locate these accurately you should count the vertebrae. As a guideline, the seventh cervical vertebra (cervical means vertebrae in the neck) is felt as a prominent bony lump where the neck joins the upper part of the back. This acts as a useful marker for the accurate localization of points on the back.

The direction of massage

We have already mentioned the idea of channels and the flow of qi or vital energy through these channels. Better results will be obtained with acupressure if the point is massaged in the direction of the flow of qi. On the diagrams, arrows are provided to guide you. The point should be massaged in the direction of the arrows. If you localize a tender point then it may be necessary to go back to the diagrams of the channels and try to work out on which channel the point lies. If it is impossible for you define the channel on which the point lies, then massage the point deeply with a vertical movement. Where several points lie close together the arrow at the head of these points gives a direction of massage for all the points.

Method and duration of massage

The amount of pressure applied should be the same in each case, but it may vary according to the type of complaint and the patient's age. In very general terms, for acute pain a larger amount of active massage should be provided. For chronic pain:

New-born babies:	½-3 minutes
Babies of 3-6 months:	1-4 minutes
Babies of 6-12 months:	1-5 minutes
Children aged 1-3:	2-7 minutes
Older children:	5-10 minutes
Adults:	5-15 minutes

The frequency of treatment depends on the type and severity

of the complaint. In general terms, you should massage the points daily or twice a day for chronic pain and up to ten times a day for very acute pain. In acute pain the more treatment given, the better the result. Sometimes you may experience a short-term worsening of the pain immediately after acupressure. This means that the treatment is almost certainly going to be effective, but too much massage has been given. In such instances the frequency and duration of treatment should be decreased.

When applying acupressure you should first massage points on the side of the pain using local and distal points. General points should be massaged bilaterally. Local and distal points can be massaged bilaterally if unilateral massage fails to produce a good result. The following general guidelines should be followed:

1. The room temperature should be comfortable, not too hot or not too cold.
2. Make sure the air is fresh, don't work in a stale or smoky atmosphere.
3. Sit or lie in a comfortable position and work with warm hands. If necessary warm your hands by rubbing them together before starting.
4. Massage should be applied with rapid movements about 50-100 times a minute.

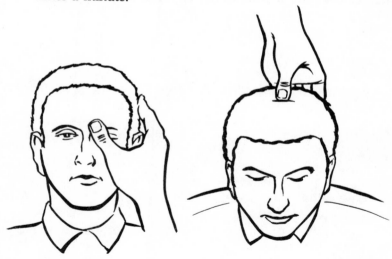

Figure 19. Acupressure must be applied by direct pressure through the tip of the thumb. These diagrams taken from a Chinese text illustrate the exact method.

5. If the patient has a sensitive skin, a little massage oil or talcum
    powder may be useful.
6. Some patients sweat freely after treatment. In such situations
    use less massage on the next treatment and remember to wrap
    up warmly on cold or windy days.
7. Do not use points Large Intestine 4 (LI4) and Spleen 6 (Sp6)
    during pregnancy. (*See Figure 23.*)

The technique of acupressure
Use the nail and tip of your index finger, massaging the points in
the direction suggested. The fingernail should be approximately
at right angles to the skin but should not damage the skin when
massaging. Massage the skin in short strokes, approximately an
inch long. The pressure on the points of the body should be strong
enough to be clearly felt — remember the point must be stimulated,
but not so strongly that it produces severe pain or bruising. The
pressure should be such that the skin becomes a little reddened
after about half a minute, but the skin surface itself must not be
injured. If you are over the correct point a deep numbing or burning
sensation may be felt. The Chinese call this 'deqi' or 'obtaining qi'.
If this sensation is obtained it is a good sign and usually means
that acupressure is likely to be very effective.

5. How to Use a TNS Machine

Transcutaneous Nerve Stimulation (TNS)
We would remind the reader again that, PAIN IS A SYMPTOM
AND A CLEAR DIAGNOSIS OF ITS CAUSE IS ESSENTIAL.
We have already defined TNS and described its probable
physiological mechanisms, and its potential adverse reactions are
discussed in the latter part of this chapter. The most important
question left unanswered about it is, 'When should you choose
TNS rather than acupressure?' We would suggest the following
guidelines:
1.   When TNS is recommended by your doctor, physiotherapist
     or any other medical or paramedical adviser.
2.   When acupressure fails to produce a sustained result. If you
     have been using acupressure for a few weeks and it only gives
     very short-term pain relief then TNS can be a very valuable
     method of increasing the duration of clinical response.
3.   If you have a TNS machine available to you, then it's probably
     better to use acupressure for acute pain and TNS for more
     chronic, long-term pain.

Usually, if TNS is going to produce a useful clinical result, you
will have noted some improvement from acupressure. However,
TNS sometimes works when acupressure fails and vice versa. It
is therefore worthwhile trying both these techniques before rejecting
this approach to pain management.

The actual use of TNS may be inconvenient; for instance, you
may not wish to use the machine while operating heavy machinery
such as a lawnmower, or while at a business meeting. In these
situations TNS can be used in the evening or when convenient,
and acupressure at other more suitable times during the day. It
is quite acceptable and sensible to combine both these approaches
to pain.

The methods for point localization for TNS are exactly the same as those used for acupressure. These are described in detail on page 49. TNS pads are usually about one inch square so point location need not be quite so exact as for acupressure, but the skin pad must be placed so that the current goes through the point needing therapy.

Choosing the right points for TNS

In pain the point most in need of treatment is the tender point. These point(s) must be considered for use in each treatment session. It is essential to choose points ONLY after referring to the relevant section on the site or diagnosis of pain, as the diagrams and descriptions will provide the detailed information required for effective treatment. The following guidelines should be borne in mind when choosing TNS as a therapy:

1. As a general principle start off with the local tender point on or around the site of pain and then, if these do not prove effective, use points further away from the pain, such as distal points.

Figure 20.

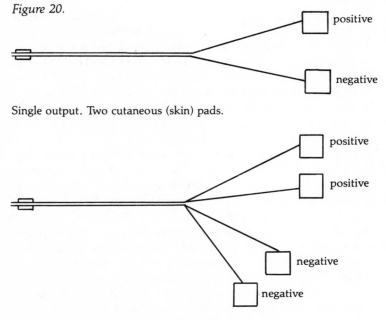

Single output. Two cutaneous (skin) pads.

Single output. Four cutaneous (skin) pads.

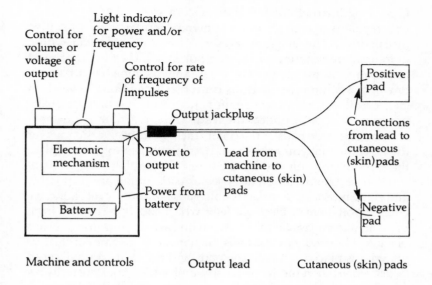

Figure 21. Diagrammatic representation of a single output TNS machine.

2. There may be a number of painful areas. Treat the most painful area first and then reassess the situation after about half an hour or so. You may find, as with acupressure, that when the most tender point has been treated all the other areas of pain disappear.

3. General points:
In the sections on each specific disease, general points are marked where applicable. These should be used at each treatment and *stimulated bilaterally*.

4. Most commercially available TNS machines have one or two outputs through which the cutaneous pads can be connected. Each output can provide two or four cutaneous pads. (See *Figure 20*.)

As a general rule, it is valuable to have equipment available so that you can treat four areas at one time. As the diagram demonstrates, this can be achieved with a slightly cheaper single output machine and a 'split lead'. Alternatively a more expensive dual output machine can be used which can, in theory, provide eight pads. It is rarely necessary to use eight pads; four should be perfectly adequate.

Operating instructions for TNS machines

When you first get the machine, unwrap it and read the operating instructions. The diagram (*Figure 21*) will provide you with a graphic representation of the components and controls of most common TNS machines. Make sure the machine has a battery; one of the commonest reasons for a machine failing to work or 'breaking down', is the fact that the battery is too low or occasionally not present at all! Connect the lead, to the machine at one end, and the electrode pads at the other; the operating instructions for the machine that you have should explain this simply. Then place the pads on the site you have chosen to stimulate.

There are many different types of pads, some are disposable and some reusable. The disposable pads are usually self-adhesive and have on them an electrode jelly, which allows the current from the machine to pass on to the skin with ease. If your machine has black, rubberized reusable pads, then make sure some conductive material is placed between the pads and the skin. You will need to use electro-conductive jelly, some of which is almost always supplied with the machine. If you do not use the jelly then the pads may not make contact or may produce an area of skin irritation. The rubberized reusable pads invariably need some method of attaching them to the skin. This can be achieved either with elastoplast or some of the special tapes that are usually supplied with the machine.

A whole range of TNS accessories will be available from the supplier of your machine. If you have any doubts or difficulties about how to make the machine work or problems in attaching it effectively then please contact the person who has supplied your machine and ask for advice.

TNS machines have two main adjustments. One adjusts the *rate or frequency* (the number of times per second) the small packets or pulses of electricity run through the body. A graphic representation of the electrical characteristics of an individual pulse is shown in *Figure 22*. The other adjusts the *amplitude, voltage or volume* of the output itself. These two controls are labelled slightly differently on each machine, but reading the instructions thoroughly ought to clarify the situation. In general terms, high-frequency stimulation (that is more than 100 hertz or cycles per second) is useful for acute pain or when the TNS is only being used for a short period. Low-frequency stimulation (10 hertz or 10 cycles per second) is better for long-term stimulation or the more prolonged use of a TNS machine. Often the detailed frequency

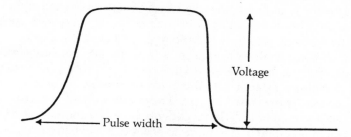

Figure 22. Diagrammatic representation of the electrical output from a typical TNS machine.

adjustments on the machine are difficult to translate into exact frequencies. However, it should be possible, on all TNS machines, to adjust them so that an output of less than 10 hertz or more than 100 hertz can be obtained.

The power or amplitude of the output should be adjusted so that a *comfortable tingling sensation is felt.* It is not necessary to cause pain with TNS as this will not improve the results obtained.

Some machines have an adjustment for pulse width. This adjustment refers to the actual width of the pulse, and is usually timed in micro-seconds. Some people find particular pulse widths uncomfortable, and others more comfortable. The machine should be adjusted so that the sensation felt is comfortable. To date there is no good evidence to suggest that variation of the pulse width will affect the outcome of treatment. Therefore, if it is to be adjusted, it should be adjusted on the basis of comfort alone.

Most TNS machines take small 9 volt PP3 batteries. These can easily be bought in almost any garage or corner shop. If the machine is to be used daily, for prolonged periods of time (ten or fifteen hours a day), then it may be much cheaper to buy rechargeable nickel-cadmium batteries, rather than continuing to use two or three disposable batteries every week.

General guidelines for the use of TNS machines
There are a number of general guidelines for the use of TNS which all those wishing to use the machines will find valuable to consider:
1. It is useful to borrow a machine for a few weeks before deciding to purchase one. In this way its effectiveness can be assessed and you can decide whether purchasing a machine is really worthwhile.

2. The machine should initially be used for between half an hour and an hour every day. You may find that increased use of the machine produces increased pain relief. If this does occur then the machine can be used for prolonged periods during the day — some patients find that they need to use it for twenty-four hours a day. Using the machine continuously does not necessarily decrease its effect. The requirements for particular types of pain or individual patients vary enormously, and the machine should be used so as to produce the maximum clinical benefit.

3. Locate the negative or black electrode (this is usually marked on the leads in some way) over the area of greatest pain as this certainly produces increased benefit. It is not necessary to consider the course, distribution or flow of the channels when using TNS machines.

4. The easiest people from whom to borrow machines are doctors, physiotherapists and pain clinics.

Clinical response

During the two- or three-week experimental period the machine should be tried, in rotation, on all the points suggested for the treatment of each specific disease, as described in Chapter 6. The frequency and duration of treatment ought to be varied, until the patient decides on the 'best' combination for the pain. The most critical variable is the exact location of the electrode pads, small changes in the positioning of the pads may give a vast improvement in response. The patient must therefore pay close attention to the diagrams and point locations suggested so that the pads are placed over the acupuncture points.

During this three or four weeks one of four clinical responses may occur:

1. You may notice *swift and immediate improvement*. In such instances you may find the TNS machine needs to be used infrequently (perhaps once every three or four days) in order to produce a good clinical response.

2. *A slow but sure response*. You may notice gradually increasing pain relief over the initial two or three weeks; the pain relief obtained may go on improving for up to six or nine months but is then likely to stabilize. If this sort of response is obtained the machine should be used frequently and regularly as the more treatment you give the better the response.

3. Some patients notice *a reaction to treatment*. This means that

the pain may become temporarily worse after treatment; if such a reaction occurs then it's highly likely a good response will be obtained from TNS, if the machine is used for short, infrequent periods. A reaction means you have over-treated yourself.

4. You may notice *no improvement*. If no change in your pain occurs after three or four weeks of using TNS at the different frequencies and at different sites on the body then we suggest you abandon this technique, as it is unlikely to prove of long-term value for your pain.

These instructions really demand that a TNS machine should be in the patient's possession throughout the three or four week trial period. Some doctors and physiotherapists only use the machine for short periods during the week or may only lend machines for a week or so at a time. This represents an inadequate trial of TNS as a more prolonged and diligent approach to this technique may often produce results when an initial 'go' of an hour or two has failed.

Adverse reactions

TNS is a very safe technique, particularly if the ensuing advice is followed.

1. DO NOT TREAT PAIN WITHOUT KNOWING ITS CAUSE. PAIN IS A SYMPTOM THAT DEMANDS A DIAGNOSIS. IT MAY BE DANGEROUS TO TREAT PAIN WITHOUT AN ADEQUATE DIAGNOSIS.

2. Do not use TNS machines if you have a pacemaker. Occasionally the rhythm of a heart pacemaker may be dangerously modified by a TNS machine. It is perfectly safe to use a TNS machine if somebody in your family or standing next to you has a pacemaker; it is just that you should not use the machine if you have a pacemaker.

3. Occasionally a skin reaction to the electrode jelly may be noticed. It is frequently an itchy rash which gets worse on contact with the gel. If you notice this, change the gel. If it becomes persistent then seek medical advice as simple creams will often settle this reaction. You should also consider the use of different sites for electrode placement.

4. If you are pregnant please avoid using points LI4 and Sp6. (See *Figure 23*.)

5. It could be hazardous to use a TNS machine while operating heavy machinery such as a car or a lawnmower or while

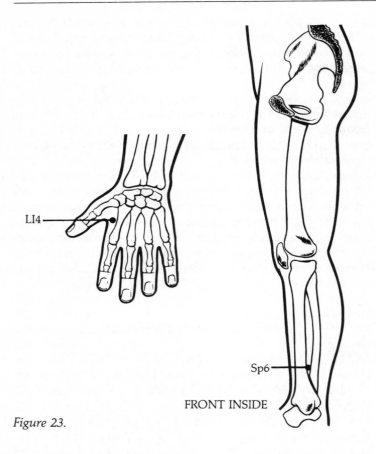

LI4

Sp6

FRONT INSIDE

Figure 23.

cooking. Occasionally you may accidentally adjust the amplitude button so that you receive a sudden electric shock; this could precipitate the car or lawnmower going out of control or a hot cooking pot being spilled over someone else. Therefore, if at all possible, do not use TNS machines in situations which are likely to be at risk from this type of hazard.

Choosing and obtaining your machine

It is possible to obtain TNS machines without going through a doctor, physiotherapist or any other medical worker but we would not advise this. TNS is a technique that is now widely used by the medical profession and it should be quite possible for you to approach your general practitioner or physiotherapist in order to discuss the advisability of using this technique. They may well have a machine they can lend you for the first two to three weeks to see if it helps, prior to your needing to purchase one.

Machines vary in price enormously, from about £20 to £500. The clinical effectiveness and electrical characteristics of the machines vary slightly, but not in any major way. The price variation represents, largely, differences in packaging and marketing techniques rather than any innate therapeutic superiority. It is therefore wise to choose a middle range machine, that is likely to stand relatively heavy use, but is not over-expensive. The sort of target price we feel you should be aiming for is between £50 and £80 for a single output machine and £70 to £120 for a machine with two outputs. The three largest manufacturers and distributors of TNS machines in the United Kingdom are: Spembly Medical Limited, Newbury Road, Andover, Hampshire, SP10 4DR; Neen Pain Products, Barn Lodge, Gooseberry Hill, Swanton Morley, Dereham, Norfolk, NR20 4NR; RDG Electro-Medical Equipment, 429 Brighton Road, Croydon, Surrey, CR2 6UD. The machines produced by these three companies are illustrated on page 26 and 27.

Although there is good evidence that these machines provide a great deal of pain relief, and can often be used to diminish or replace the number of pain-killing medications required, the Department of Health has not yet made TNS available on prescription. Occasionally pain clinics, charities or physiotherapy departments may be able to let you have these machines on a long loan. However, as a general rule you should assume that you will need to purchase a TNS machine if you want to use it for a prolonged time.

If your doctor or physiotherapist is prepared to sign a form saying that you need the machine because of a chronic complaint then you will not have to pay VAT on its purchase price. This is another good reason for approaching your doctor or physiotherapist when you are thinking about purchasing a TNS machine, as their support will save you money.

6. Treatment of Specific Diseases

General guidelines
The following general guidelines should be followed in the treatment of pain, whether it be by acupressure or TNS.

1. Please read Chapter 4 on how to apply acupressure before using acupressure and Chapter 5 on how to apply TNS before using TNS.

2. Make sure that you know what is causing the pain before you begin to treat it. Pain is a symptom which may be a warning sign; YOU SHOULD ALWAYS HAVE A DIAGNOSIS FOR YOUR PAIN, FROM A COMPETENT MEDICAL PRACTITIONER, BEFORE INITIATING TREATMENT.

3. In the treatment of pain it is important to start by treating local points on or around the site of pain.

4. When treating a painful area examine the area with care and define the most painful local point. This should be treated first. You may well need a friend or relative to help with either acupressure or TNS if the painful point is out of reach, for instance on the back.

5. If you find a tender point that is not shown on the diagrams pertaining to each disease, then it should be treated. The Chinese call this the Ah Shi or 'ouch' point. The Ah Shi point should always be treated in any painful condition.

6. You should then treat distal (distant) points. Local and distal points should ideally be treated for almost all conditions at each treatment session. In some cases distal points are not required, but this is described clearly in the sections on diseases that follow.

7. Some of the diseases will also include the treatment of general points. These points act to provide general tonification and will help improve the results obtained by acupressure and TNS.

Headache (migraine) occipital

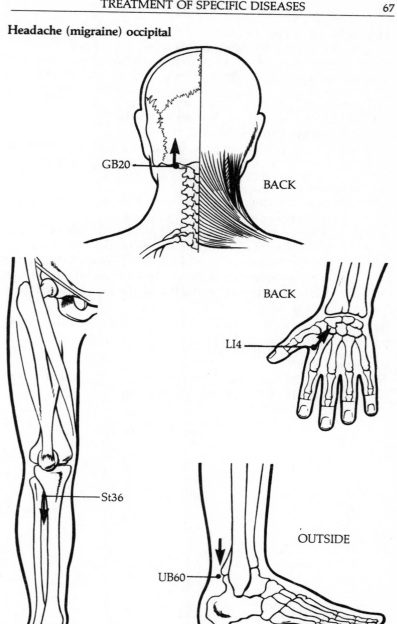

BACK

BACK

FRONT

OUTSIDE

Headache (migraine) temple

This is a headache occurring on the side of the head.

Point locations

a) Local points:

GB20   At the bottom of the back of the skull just next to the top vertebra of the neck.

Taiyang This is over the temple, in the muscles just behind the eye, but on the same level as the outer part of the eye.

b) Distal points:

SJ5   About 4 cm up from the back of the wrist between the two prominent bones of the forearm.

GB34   About 6 cm below the knee joint, on the side of the leg. Just below the bony prominence on the side of the leg.

UB60   On the lateral aspect of the ankle. Midway between the bony prominence of the ankle joint and the tendon at the back of the leg, in the thin fleshy area between these two Bandmarks.

Liv3   About 5cm above the crease between the first and second toes.

c) General point:

St36   About 7 cm down from the bottom of the knee cap and 2 cm lateral to the crest of the shin.

Headache (migraine) temple

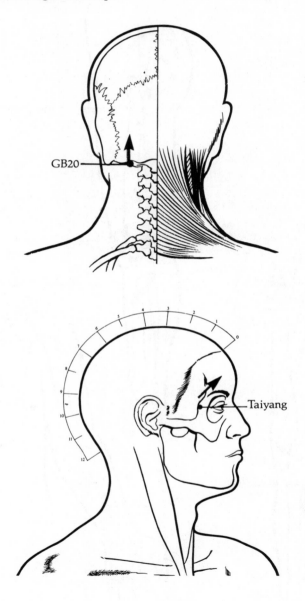

Headache (migraine) temple

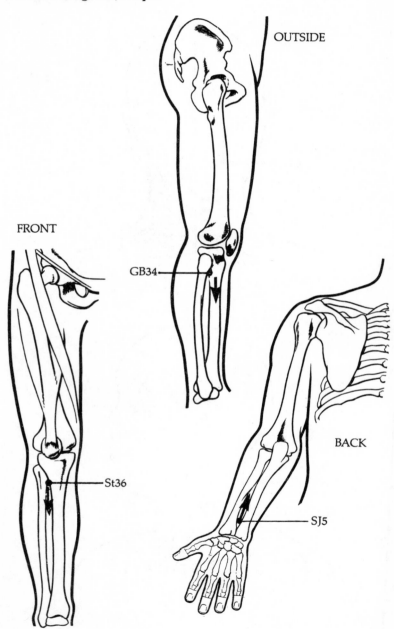

OUTSIDE

FRONT

GB34

St36

BACK

SJ5

Headache (migraine) temple

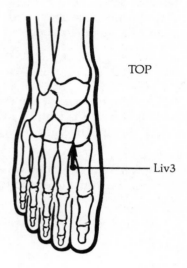

TOP

Liv3

OUTSIDE

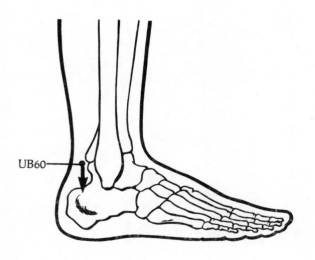

UB60

Eye pain

This can occur for a whole variety of reasons. It is most commonly associated with headaches and migraine, but if you have persistent eye pain that is not associated with headaches then please seek the opinion of a qualified doctor or ophthalmic optician.

Point locations

a) Local points:

UB1   The inner corner of the eye.

Taiyang This is over the temple, in the muscles just behind the eye, but on the same level as the outer part of the eye.

b) Distal point:

LI4   Between the thumb and first finger, about 2 cm down from the knuckle of the first finger.

c) General point:

Liv3   About 5 cm above the crease between the first and second toes.

Eye pain

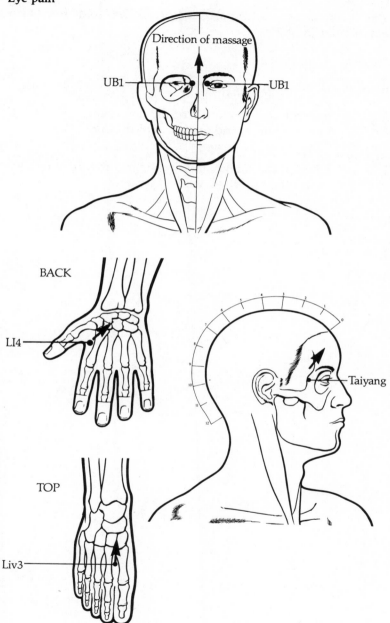

Jaw pain
This is usually caused by arthritis of the jaw joint (temporo-mandibular joint).

Point locations

a) Local points:
St6   This is right on the angle of the jaw bone.
St7   Just in front of and below the jaw joint.
SI19   Just in front of and almost over the ear canal.

b) Distal point:
LI4   Between the thumb and first finger, about 2 cm down
         from the knuckle of the first finger.

Jaw pain

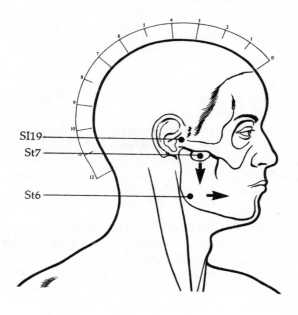

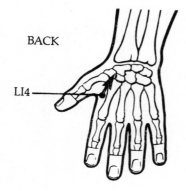

Toothache

If you have a toothache then there is probably a good dental reason for it and you should consult your dentist for an opinion. Acupressure and TNS may be used to alleviate the acute pain.

Point locations

a) Local points:

St7   (For the treatment of dental pain in the upper jaw.)
       Just in front of and below the jaw joint.

St6   (For the treatment of dental pain in the lower jaw.)
       This is right on the angle of the jaw bone.

Remember to treat points on the side of the pain and treat any tender points by massaging or connecting your TNS machine over the area of pain on the face.

b) Distal points:

St44   (For the treatment of dental pain in the upper jaw.)
       This point is to be found 1 cm up from the web separating the second and third toes.

LI4   (For the treatment of dental pain in the lower jaw.)
       Between the thumb and first finger, about 2 cm down from the knuckle of the first finger.

Toothache

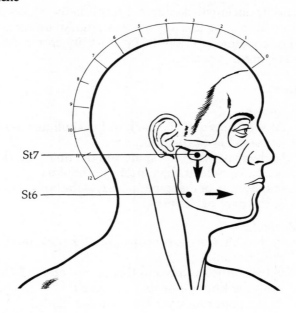

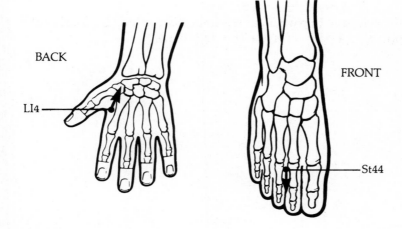

BACK

FRONT

Neck pain

Chronic neck pain is usually due to arthritis in the neck, but acute neck pain may be due to a sprain or strain. An opinion from a qualified osteopathic or chiropractic practitioner may be of real value in helping this problem.

Point locations

a) Local points:

GB20   At the bottom of the back of the skull just next to the top vertebra of the neck.

GB21   Midway between the spine and the tip of the shoulder, on the muscle at the top of the shoulder.

Du14   In the centre of the spine just below the bony prominence at the base of the neck.

b) Distal points:

LI4   (If the pain runs over the front of the neck and the front of the shoulder.)
       Between the thumb and first finger, about 2 cm down from the knuckle of the first finger.

SI3   (If the pain runs over the shoulder blade.)
       At the base of the little finger, just underneath the knuckle of the little finger. When using massage, place your thumb on the palmar surface of the hand and massage down towards the wrist.

In neck pain, in particular, it is important to look for local tender points especially over the shoulder blade.

Neck pain

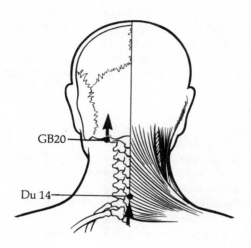

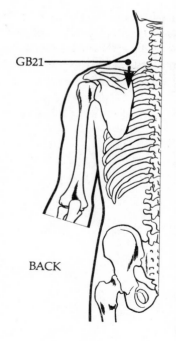

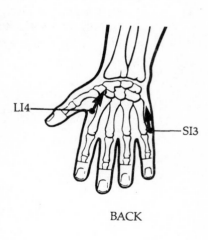

Shoulder pain
Shoulder pain should be treated early and vigorously. If shoulder pain is allowed to become chronic then a frozen shoulder may develop in which pain and limited movement may be present for a year or two. If you are not getting a quick result with treatment then seek an opinion from a doctor or physiotherapist.

Point locations

a) Local points:

GB21   Midway between the spine and the tip of the shoulder, on the muscle at the top of the shoulder.

LI14   About 5 cm below the front of the armpit, on the side of the shoulder.

LI15   On the front of the shoulder, just below the crest of the bone overhanging the shoulder joint.

SJ14   On the back of the shoulder, just below the crest of the bone overhanging the shoulder joint.

b) Distal point:

LI11   On the lateral aspect of the elbow, in the fleshy muscle midway between the elbow joint and the elbow crease.

LI4   If pain is radiating down the arm use this point. Between the thumb and first finger, about 2cm down from the knuckle of the first finger.

Shoulder pain

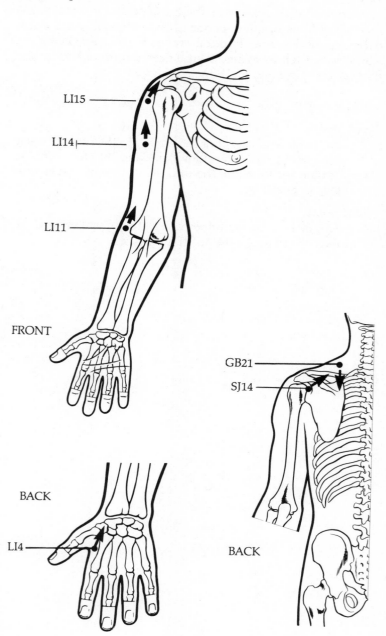

LI15

LI14

LI11

FRONT

BACK

LI4

GB21

SJ14

BACK

Tennis elbow

This is due to inflammation of the muscles that insert into the humerus (the bone of the upper arm) and extend down the arm into the back of the hand. If the elbow has been strained with too much activity such as tennis, then inflammation of the tendon (muscular insertion into the bone) results.

Point locations

a) Local point:

LI11   On the lateral aspect of the elbow, in the fleshy muscle midway between the elbow joint and the elbow crease.

It is very important to define the local tender point and treat it as accurately as possible.

b) Distal point:

SJ5   About 4 cm up from the back of the wrist between the two prominent bones of the forearm.

Tennis elbow

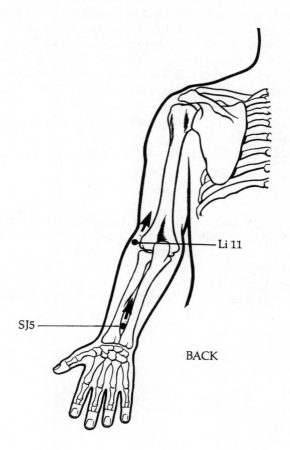

Li 11

SJ5

BACK

Wrist pain

This is most frequently caused by a strain to the wrist produced
by over-use. It is commonly found in people who suddenly do
a lot of activity such as gardening in the first few weeks of the
spring and in some patients with rheumatoid arthritis. Occasionally
a nerve travelling through the wrist and into the hand may be
'trapped' at the wrist. This is called a carpal tunnel syndrome and
may give rise to pain in the wrist and arm, particularly at night.
Wrist pain may also be associated with arthritis of the neck, and
nerves trapped in the neck may cause pain to radiate down into
the wrist and hand.

Only local points need to be used to treat wrist pain.

Point locations

Local points:

P7	This is in the middle of the palmar aspect of the wrist. It is particularly useful for carpal tunnel syndrome.
SJ4	The middle of the back of the wrist.
SI5	On the back, little finger side of the wrist, just where the hand joins the wrist.
LI5	At the base of the thumb where it joins the wrist.

Wrist pain

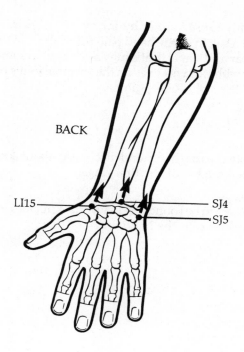

BACK

LI15   SJ4
     SJ5

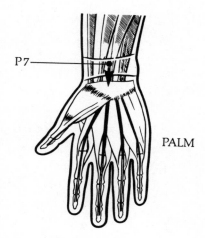

P7

PALM

Hand pain
This is usually caused either by injury or arthritis. Rheumatoid arthritis will result in severe hand pain particularly in the mornings, osteo- or wear and tear arthritis may also result in some hand pain, particularly with extra nodules on the terminal joints of the fingers. You should use only local points.

Point location

a) Local point:
LI4   Between the thumb and first finger, about 2cm down from the knuckle of the first finger.

b) Extra points:
These points are to be found just below the knuckles in the muscles between the bones in the hand.

Hand pain

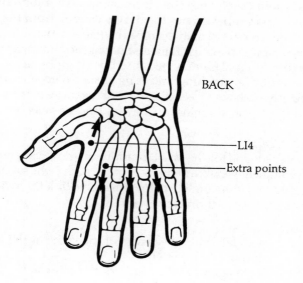

BACK

LI4

Extra points

Intercostal neuralgia
This is pain usually resulting from arthritis or injury to the spine; this injury in turn irritates the nerves coming from the spine and can result in pain radiating from the back to the side or front. It is important to diagnose the cause of pain accurately as sometimes intercostal neuralgia may be caused by shingles, heart disease or an infection in the lung and lung tissue. Before treatment it is imperative to have a clear diagnosis of the cause of the pain. When treating the pain, examine carefully for tender points and treat these.

Point locations
When searching for the point locations on the back remember that the prominent vertebra at the base of the neck is the seventh cervical vertebra and immediately below this is the first thoracic vertebra. There are twelve thoracic vertebrae.

a) Local points:

UB12	4cm lateral to the centre of the spine at the level of the 2nd thoracic vertebra.
UB13	4 cm lateral to the centre of the spine at the level of the 3rd thoracic vertebra.
UB14	4cm lateral to the centre of the spine at the level of the 4th thoracic vertebra.
UB15	4cm lateral to the centre of the spine at the level of the 5th thoracic vertebra.
UB16	4cm lateral to the centre of the spine at the level of the 6th thoracic vertebra.
UB17	4cm lateral to the centre of the spine at the level of the 7th thoracic vertebra.
UB18	4cm lateral to the centre of the spine at the level of the 9th thoracic vertebra.
UB19	4cm lateral to the centre of the spine at the level of the 10th thoracic vertebra.

b) Distal points:

GB34	About 6cm below the knee joint, on the side of the leg. Just below the bony prominence on the side of the leg.
Liv3	5cm above the crease between the first and second toes.

Intercostal neuralgia

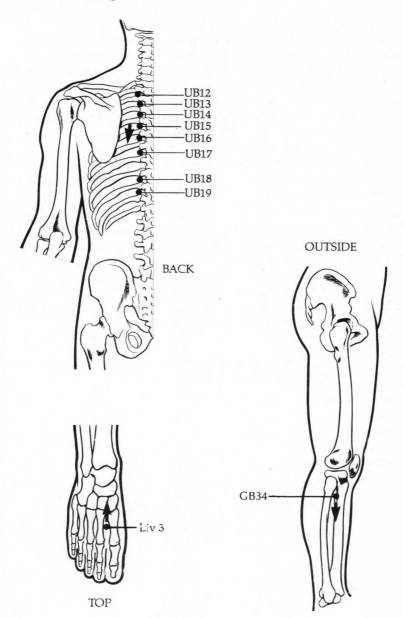

UB12
UB13
UB14
UB15
UB16
UB17
UB18
UB19

BACK

OUTSIDE

GB34

Liv 3

TOP

Back pain

Back pain is most commonly due to arthritis affecting the back narrowing the discs that separate the five lumbar vertebral bodies. Occasionally it can be due to a slipped or prolapsed intervertebral disc. In such cases the pain often extends down the leg causing sciatica. If you have severe back pain which does not respond satisfactorily to acupressure or TNS it may well be a prolapsed disc, and a competent osteopathic, chiropractic or orthopaedic opinion should then be sought. A very small proportion of prolapsed intervertebral discs require surgical intervention and subsequent removal of the protruding disc.

It is important to localize and treat the tender points in back pain.

Point locations

a) Local points:

UB25   About 4 cm lateral to the centre of the spine at the level of the junction of the 4th and 5th lumbar vertebrae.

UB31   About 4 cm lateral to the centre of the spine, on the sacrum, just below the 5th lumbar vertebra.

If pain radiates into the buttock, use GB30.

GB30   This is in the centre of the buttock and must be massaged deeply with considerable pressure.

b) Distal point:

UB40   At the back of the knee, in the middle of the crease at the back of the knee.

Back pain

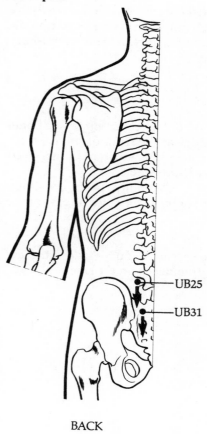

BACK

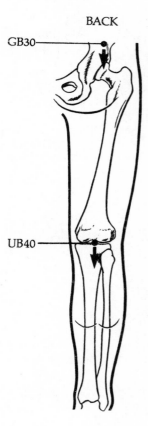

Hip pain
This is most commonly due to osteo-arthritis of the hip. If the simple treatment of acupressure or TNS fails then seek an orthopaedic opinion with a view to hip replacement. It is important to identify the local tender point and treat it.

Point locations

a) Local points:

GB29   Midway between the top of the femur (upper leg bone) and the bony prominence at the front of the pelvis.

GB30   This is in the centre of the buttock and must be massaged deeply with considerable pressure.

St31   Where a line dropped diagonally from the bony prominence at the front of the pelvis and the base of the pelvis actually meet.

b) Distal point:

GB34   About 6 cm below the knee joint, on the side of the leg. Just below the bony prominence on the side of the leg.

Hip pain

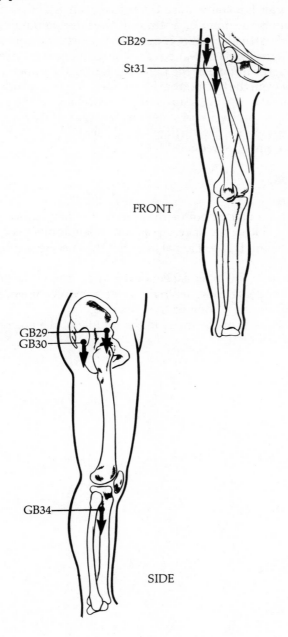

Knee pain

Chronic knee pain is usually caused by osteo-arthritis of the knee, acute knee pain by a sprain or a strain. If the knee pain remains persistent, and particularly if it is caused by a twisting injury to the joint, there may be a cartilage tear. The cartilage is a piece of gristle sitting in the middle of the joint, separating the upper long bone of the leg from the two bottom long bones. A twisting motion may tear it causing locking, pain and joint swelling. If the knee continually locks and swells because of a cartilage tear then it may be necessary to remove the cartilage surgically.

Only local points are required for the knee.

Point locations

a) Local points:

Xiyan   This is a pair of points that can be felt just below and to the side of the knee cap as soft indentations over the knee joint. It is best to palpate with the knee bent at right angles.

Sp9   This is on the inner aspect of the knee, below the knee joint and just underneath the inner bony prominence of the main long bone of the lower leg.

UB40   At the back of the knee, in the middle of the crease at the back of the knee.

Knee pain

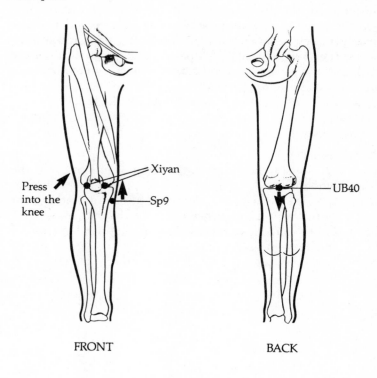

FRONT   BACK

Ankle pain

If the ankle pain is chronic it is usually due to an arthritic process, if acute it is due to a sprain or strain. Acupressure and TNS are probably the best methods of dealing with ankle sprain and arthritis affecting the ankle. In acute ankle pain you should be sure to have a medical practitioner or physiotherapist look at your ankle in case there is a small fracture present.

It is only necessary to use local points for the ankle.

Point locations

a) Local points:

St41   On top of the front of the ankle joint, between the tendons.

Sp5   On the inner aspect of the ankle, just below and in front of the bony prominence of the ankle joint.

GB40   On the outside of the ankle, just below and in front of the bony prominence.

Sp5 and GB40 are exactly 'opposite' each other.

Ankle pain

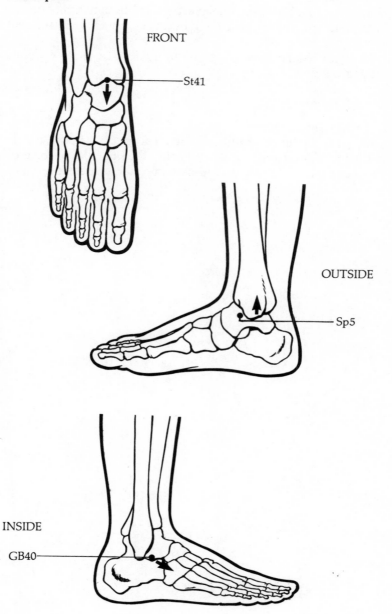

FRONT

St41

OUTSIDE

Sp5

INSIDE

GB40

Foot pain
Pain in the foot is usually due to arthritis although it may be due
to an acute sprain or strain caused by an event such as an accident
or sport.

Only use local points, and examine the foot carefully to define
these accurately.

Point locations

a) Local points:
Only treat the tender points. There are a group of 'extra points'
in the foot. These are found just behind the knuckles of the toes,
between the bones and in the muscle tissue that separates the bones.

Foot pain

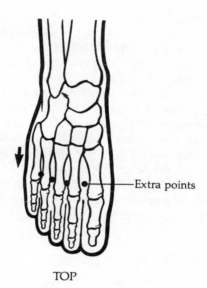

Extra points

TOP

Sciatica

Sciatica is simply a descriptive term used to define pain travelling down the sciatic nerve. The sciatic nerve runs from the low back down the leg to the foot. Sciatica is usually caused by arthritis in the low back which results in pressure on the nerves as they travel down the spine. It may also be caused by small anatomical 'dislocations' in the many joints between the vertebrae. This means that sciatica may be helped by spinal manipulation if it does not respond to either acupressure or TNS. Very occasionally severe sciatica may result from a prolapsed intervertebral disc. If the problem is severe and does not settle spontaneously over a two- or three-month period then it may be necessary to have an operation to remove the disc; such operations are very rarely required and should only be considered seriously if the pain is severe, persistent and has been present for some months.

Point locations

a) Local points:

GB30   This is in the centre of the buttock and must be massaged deeply with considerable pressure.

UB31   About 4 cm lateral to the centre of the spine, on the sacrum, just below the 5th lumbar vertebra.

UB32   About 2 cm below UB31, perpendicularly underneath it.

UB33   About 2 cm below UB32, perpendicularly underneath it.

b) Distal points:

UB37   On the back of the thigh, in the middle of a line joining GB30 and UB40.

UB40   At the back of the knee, in the middle of the crease at the back of the knee.

UB57   In the middle of the back of the calf. Midway on a line joining UB40 and UB60.

UB60   On the lateral aspect of the ankle. Midway between the bony prominence of the ankle joint and the tendon at the back of the leg, in the thin fleshy area between these two landmarks.

If pain is down the side of the leg:

GB34   About 6 cm below the knee joint, on the side of the leg. Just below the bony prominence on the side of the leg.

Sciatica

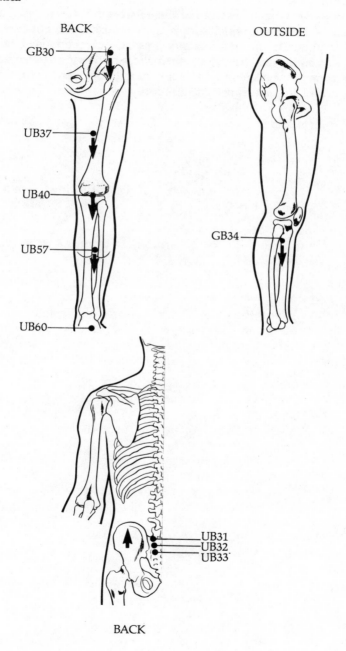

Cramp

Cramp may be due to spasm of the muscles in the leg or to spasm of the blood vessels which supply the leg muscles. Treatment may work while the cramp is actually present, but it can also be used to avoid cramp occurring. If cramp in the leg seems to be precipitated recurrently by exercise, such as walking 100 metres, then it is important to seek a medical opinion.

Point locations

a) Local points:

UB40   At the back of the knee, in the middle of the crease at the back of the knee.

UB57   In the middle of the back of the calf. Midway on a line joining UB40 and UB60.

b) General points:

P6   On the inside of the arm, 4 cm from the wrist crease.

Cramp

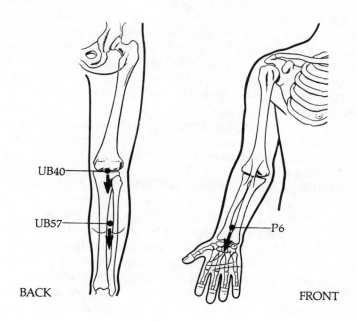

UB40

UB57

BACK

P6

FRONT

Shingles

This is an infection due to the Herpes Zoster virus; the same virus causes Chicken Pox. It often starts with a general 'flu-like illness and then presents with a vesicular rash over the abdomen, leg or face. The rash over the abdomen is often diagonal, running from the back towards the front. This condition is particularly painful and should be treated vigorously with either acupressure or TNS. Very occasionally the pain from shingles can give rise to a chronic condition known as post-herpetic neuralgia. This is much more difficult to treat with acupressure and TNS, but these techniques may just be of benefit in helping post-herpetic neuralgia. If the acute shingles is treated vigorously then post-herpetic neuralgia can frequently be avoided.

Do not treat points on the rash itself. When using acupressure, massage all around the rash and when using TNS, use a machine with four electrodes, placing three of them around the rash randomly. If the rash remains particularly painful and does not seem to respond to this treatment, then use the normal side, directing your acupressure or TNS treatment at the mirror image pain points. In other words, treat the normal side as if it were the painful side. Active treatment on the rash itself may well make the situation much worse. It is important to treat the general points bilaterally and actively. Treatment should be repeated three or four times a day.

Point location
The illustration over the page demonstrates ringing the rash and the treatment of the opposite side.

General point:
Liv3   About 5 cm above the crease between the first and second toes.

Shingles

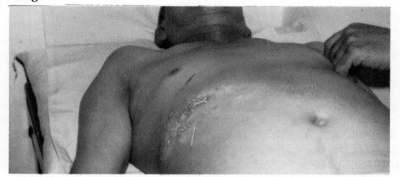

SIDE

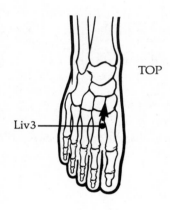

TOP

Liv3

Dysmenorrhoea

This is a common problem, particularly among young women who haven't yet had children. Dysmenorrhoea is less likely to occur after the first pregnancy. Acupressure and TNS can be used both to help acute dysmenorrhoea and prophylactically to prevent dysmenorroea occurring. If you are using it to treat acute pain then repeat the treatment every hour or two until the pain goes away. If you wish to use the points to prevent dysmenorrhoea occurring then treat every other day for the week before you are expecting a period.

All the points used have a general effect; there are no specific local points.

Point locations

UB31   About 4 cm lateral to the centre of the spine, on the sacrum, just below the fifth lumbar vertebra.

Ren6   About 3 cm below the umbilicus.

St36   About 7 cm down from the bottom of the knee cap and 2 cm lateral to the crest of the shin.

Sp6   About 7 cm above the tip of the bony prominence of the ankle. Just behind the shin bone in the muscular compartment of the leg.

Liv3   About 5 cm above the crease between the first and second toes.

Dysmenorrhoea

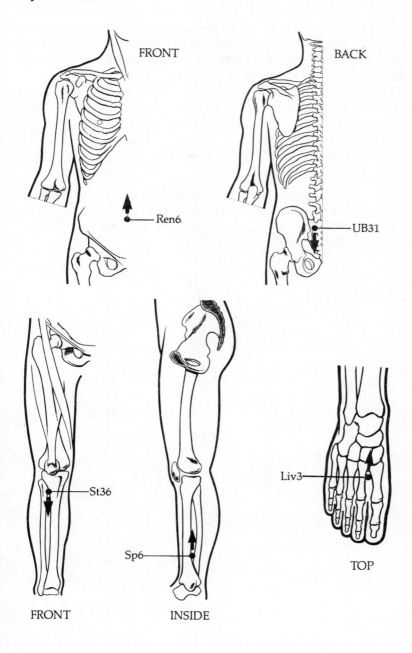

FRONT

BACK

Ren6

UB31

St36

Sp6

Liv3

FRONT

INSIDE

TOP

Renal colic
This is a pain that is caused by the passage of a hard object, usually a kidney stone, down the ureter. The ureter is the tube that connects the kidney to the bladder; the passage of the stone down the ureter can be exceptionally painful, but it is fortunately a short-lived pain which almost never becomes chronic.

Point locations

a) Local point:
UB20   About 4 cm lateral to the centre of the spine at the level of the eleventh thoracic vertebra.

b) Distal point:
K3   On the medial or inner aspect of the ankle, halfway between the prominent ankle bone and the tendon at the back of the ankle, in the soft fleshy area between the bone and the tendon.

Renal colic

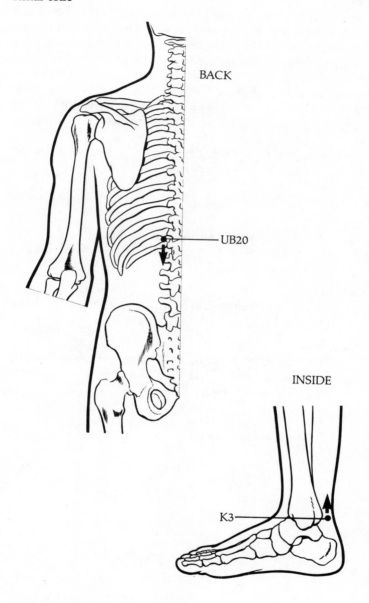

Sinusitis

Sinusitis is a very common complaint and can occur either in the maxillary sinuses which lie deep in the face below both eyes, or in the frontal sinuses which are above the eyes on either side of the bridge of the nose. People with sinusitis should consider the use of diet, and the avoidance of foods which produce excessive mucus such as milk and dairy products and red meat. Attention should also be paid to bowel function, as even slight constipation in people who are predisposed to sinusitis can lead to troublesome chronic recurrent sinusitis.

In acute sinusitis treat frequently, every few hours during the day. If the sinusitis is chronic or recurrent, treat daily.

Point locations

a) Local points:

Yintang   Between the two eyebrows, on the bridge of the nose.
LI20   Just on the side of the nose, at the level of the bottom of the nose.

b) Distal point:

LI4   Between the thumb and first finger, about 2 cm down from the knuckle of the first finger.

c) General point:

Sp6   About 7 cm above the tip of the bony prominence of the ankle. Just behind the shin bone in the muscular compartment of the leg.

Sinusitis

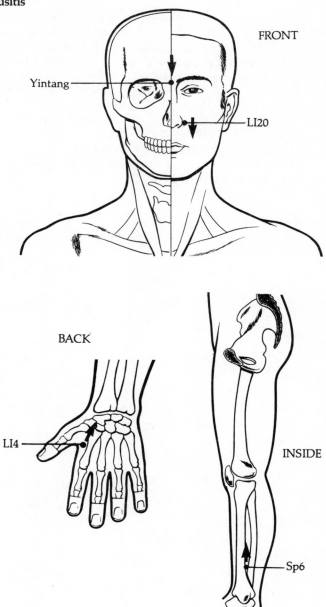

FRONT

Yintang

LI20

BACK

LI4

INSIDE

Sp6

Mouth ulcers

Mouth ulcers are a common and often troublesome complaint. It is worthwhile considering a dietary approach to mouth ulcers as some specific foods may precipitate mouth ulcers in susceptible individuals. Use general points only, treating every few hours if you have an acutely painful mouth.

Point locations

LI4   Between the thumb and first finger, about 2 cm down from the knuckle of the first finger.

St36   About 7 cm down from the bottom of the knee cap and 2 cm lateral to the crest of the shin.

Mouth ulcers

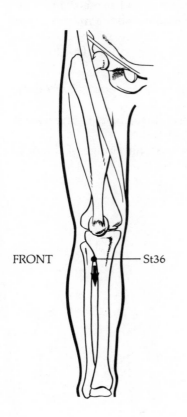

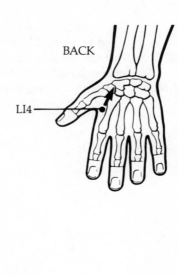

Colds and catarrh

Acupressure is a particularly useful method of shortening the natural history of cold symptoms. Treatment should be every hour or two until the cold has abated.

Point locations

LI4   Between the thumb and first finger, about 2 cm down from the knuckle of the first finger.

LI20   Just on the side of the nose, at the level of the bottom of the nose.

Yintang Between the two eyebrows, on the bridge of the nose.

Colds and catarrh

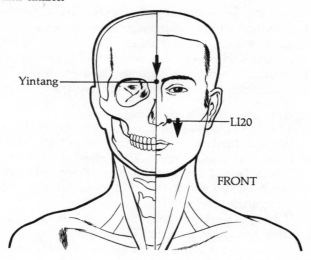

Yintang

LI20

FRONT

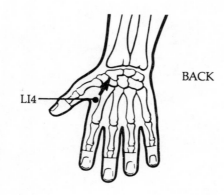

BACK

LI4

Constipation
Acupressure and TNS should only be used as supplementary therapies in people who suffer from repeated constipation. Either the diet should be changed or medical advice sought as to the cause of the constipation. However, acupressure and TNS may be useful adjuncts to therapy once the diagnosis has been made. General points are recommended, treatment should be once or twice a day.

Point locations

St36   About 7 cm down from the bottom of the knee cap and 2 cm lateral to the crest of the shin.

Sp6   About 7 cm above the tip of the bony prominence of the ankle. Just behind the shin bone in the muscular compartment of the leg.

LI4   Between the thumb and first finger, about 2 cm down from the knuckle of the first finger.

LI11   On the lateral aspect of the elbow, in the fleshy muscle midway between the elbow joint and the elbow crease.

Constipation

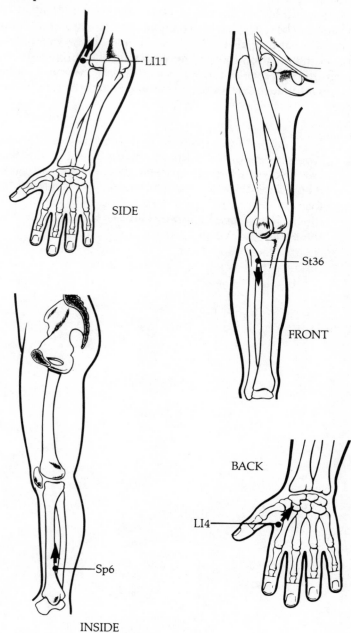

SIDE

FRONT

INSIDE

BACK

Gall-bladder colic

As with renal (kidney colic) gall-bladder colic can be particularly painful and can be relieved with a combination of acupressure and TNS. A cause for the gall-bladder colic should always be sought, as surgical intervention may be necessary to remove gall-stones or an infected gall-bladder. The points recommended should be used frequently during an acute attack and once a day if there is a low-level persistent pain.

Point locations

GB34   About 6 cm below the knee joint, on the side of the leg. Just below the bony prominence on the side of the leg.

Liv3   About 5 cm above the crease between the first and second toes.

Ren12   On the Ren channel, midway between the umbilicus and the bottom of the sternum.

Gall-bladder colic

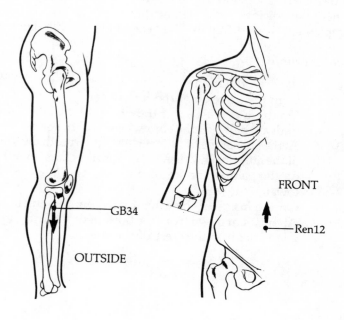

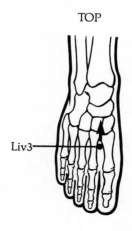

Flatulence

Flatulence frequently accompanies constipation and diarrhoea. Excessive flatulence should be managed either with dietary measures or herbal medicines. However, acupressure and TNS may act to complement these therapies. Use general points on a daily basis.

Point locations

LI4   Between the thumb and first finger, about 2 cm down from the knuckle of the first finger.

LI11   On the lateral aspect of the elbow, in the fleshy muscle midway between the elbow joint and the elbow crease.

SI3   At the base of the little finger, just underneath the knuckle of the little finger. When using massage, place your thumb on the palmar surface of the hand and massage down towards the wrist.

P6   On the inside of the arm, 4 cm from the wrist crease.

St36   About 7 cm down from the bottom of the knee cap and 2 cm lateral to the crest of the shin.

Flatulence

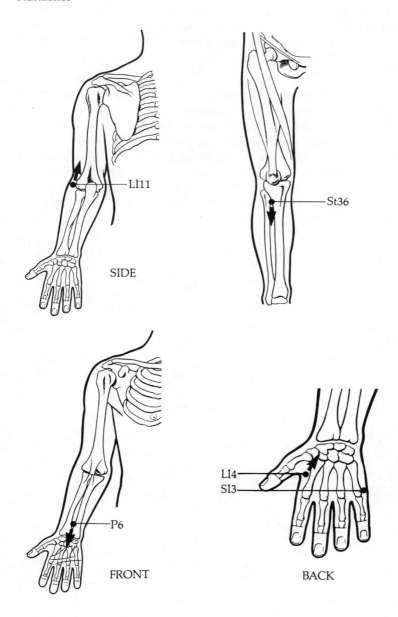

Nausea, travel sickness and early morning sickness
Acupressure and TNS are particularly good methods of relieving nausea. If the situation is acute, treat frequently until the nausea settles, every hour or so. General points only are recommended.

Point locations

P6   On the inside of the arm, 4 cm from the wrist crease.
Ren6   About 3 cm below the umbilicus.
St36   About 7 cm down from the bottom of the knee cap and 2 cm lateral to the crest of the shin.
Liv3   About 5 cm above the crease between the first and second toes.

Nausea, travel sickness and early morning sickness

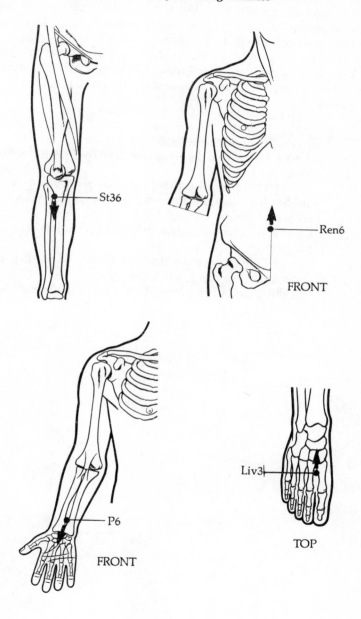

Stomach pains and stomach ulcers

If you have abdominal pain then it is essential that you see your doctor before attempting to use acupressure or TNS. However, sometimes conventional medication or surgery may not relieve all your pain immediately. In such instances, acupressure and TNS can be used as complementary therapy. General points will need to be used and treatment repeated as frequently as the pain demands.

Point locations

Liv3   About 5 cm above the crease between the first and second toes.

Sp6   About 7 cm above the tip of the bony prominence of the ankle. Just behind the shin bone in the muscular compartment of the leg.

Ren12   On the Ren channel, midway between the umbilicus and the bottom of the sternum.

St36   About 7 cm down from the bottom of the knee cap and 2 cm lateral to the crest of the shin.

P6   On the inside of the arm, 4 cm from the wrist crease.

Stomach pains and stomach ulcers

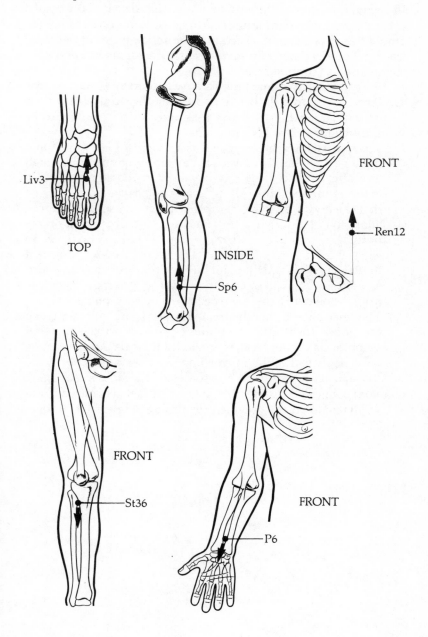

Liv3

TOP

INSIDE

Sp6

FRONT

Ren12

FRONT

St36

FRONT

P6

Phantom limb pain

Phantom limb pain is the pain or spasm that occasionally results after a limb has been amputated. The commonest reasons for amputation are a trauma, such as a car accident, or, in the older age group, vascular problems resulting in decreased blood supply to the affected limb.

When treating phantom limb pain two approaches can be used:

1. If there are particularly tender areas on the stump of the limb or digit, then these can be massaged with acupressure or stimulated with a TNS machine.
2. The normal limb can be treated as if it were the phantom limb. If we assume that there has been an amputation at mid-thigh level after a car accident, this may result in phantom ankle pain in the amputated limb. The phantom pain is caused by the fact that the body still has a 'complete' image of itself and cannot adapt to the idea that a limb has been lost. Treatment on the normal leg should use either acupressure or TNS on the good leg as if the good leg had pain. Therefore in ankle pain, treat the tender points and the points around the ankle recommended on page 96. You will often notice that the pain may disappear from the phantom ankle and be present over the phantom knee. The knee should then be treated in the same manner, using the good knee. Pain may then progress to the level of amputation; again treatment should then be directed at the good leg, treating the mirror image tender points.

Although acupressure can be a successful method of managing phantom pain, TNS is preferable. It is quite often necessary to have a TNS machine on the good leg for prolonged periods of time.

SECTION III

7. Self-Help Techniques In Pain Management

The following chapters contain detailed descriptions of a number of techniques which can be used in the management of pain. All the techniques are similar in that they are designed to produce a state of deep physical and mental quietness. In this state our capacity to influence what is happening in our bodies seems to be enhanced.

Several different techniques are described. This is because different methods will suit different people. For example, although it is usual for mental and physical relaxation to occur together, it is not always the case. Some people can become totally physically relaxed very readily, but still be a prey to anxious, rushing thoughts. Others can attain a calm and peaceful inner state while retaining a degree of physical tension. We also differ in the ease with which we can achieve a deeply relaxed state. For some people, it is an easy natural attribute; others find it needs a lot of determined work. In addition, some of us visualize things easily, others do not. Try picturing a familiar room which you are not in at present. Is it clear to you, including the colours, and is it full of detail? Do you see pictures in your mind when you listen to music or to a radio play? Visualizers and non-visualizers might find different techniques suit them. You will be able to choose the best method for you.

As a rough guide, if you are someone who tends to express tension physically, by tensing your jaw or shoulders for example, or twitching or picking with your fingers, progressive muscular relaxation should suit you. It may be enough on its own, or you might find that your mind is not quiet even when your body is. Then, if that is the case, add another method to it. Visual imagery perhaps, if you are a visualizer, or mantra meditation if you are not. If your mind is habitually very busy, use a more complex mental exercise.

If you relax physically as soon as you sit down, or you can snuggle into bed and go straight to sleep, and muscular aches and pains are not known to you, you will not need to do the physical exercises, but could go straight into one of the contemplative techniques.

Remember that all these methods involve learning. It takes time and practice to perfect them. The first time you try any psychological technique you will probably, but not necessarily, feel good afterwards. However, you are aiming for much more than a brief period of an enhanced sense of well-being. As you go on practising, every day, you should find that you relax more readily and more deeply. The maximum effect and control may take four to six weeks of regular practice, but from the beginning you should feel that you are making progress. If, after the first week of daily practice, you are still finding it difficult to attain the desired state of relaxation and, in particular, if your attention keeps wandering, try an alternative technique. Do give each technique a reasonable trial however, as nothing can be gained by dabbling around aimlessly between them. For success, first try to choose the right technique for the kind of person you are, and then work at it systematically and regularly until you become very skilled.

Pain management

The children's book, *When The Porcupine Moved In,** is the story of a friendly and easy-going rabbit who lived a very comfortable life until the day a porcupine invited himself to stay. The porcupine took over the rabbit's bed, forcing him to sleep on a hard cot. He took the rabbit's favourite easy chair, relegating his host to a footstool. He objected to the rabbit going to social functions, and from time to time invited various prickly relatives in who completely took over the rabbit's house and his life. If the rabbit tried to confront his guest, the porcupine became alarmingly angry and bristled all over. The rabbit became ill and depressed.

The tale of the porcupine and the rabbit is an excellent analogy for chronic pain. The uninvited and unpleasant guest who forced his host into discomfort, diminution of his normal activity and depression, behaved just like pain behaves. Giving in to it made life less and less bearable. Confronting it hurt.

What the rabbit did in the end was to indulge in a burst of lateral thinking (or low animal cunning, or a psychological management technique called 'counter-conditioning', depending on your

---

* Cora Annett, *When the Porcupine Moved In* (Franklin Watts Ltd, 1972).

viewpoint). Because he knew that the porcupine would disagree with everything he suggested, he began to suggest the opposite of what he really wanted to do. He rejoiced in the hard cot and the footstool, thanking the porcupine for taking over the easy chair and bed. The porcupine became confused and paranoid and moved out.

Real life, alas, is not as simple as the happy-ever-after ending of a children's story, but the principle the rabbit used was a good one. He learned to manage the problem. He could not defeat the porcupine by aggressive confrontation or by compliance — these only made things worse. He could, however, out-think him. Using psychological management techniques for pain is much the same. It is a question of thinking, knowing your enemy, and edging it out of the centre and crown of your life, so that you can get on with living. Like the porcupine, the pain may move out, or it may skulk in a corner, or come and go, but it need not dominate you and all your life.

How?

How then is pain to be managed? There is a substantial body of evidence, from scientific research and from personal accounts, which demonstrates that the state of mind can exert a powerful influence on the perception of pain. At a very simple level, if we expect that something will hurt, or are afraid that it might, we are pre-setting ourselves to perceive pain, and it probably *will* hurt. Anticipatory anxiety enhances pain intensity. Conversely, we may tolerate a pain-producing situation better, and feel less pain, when we feel confident and calm about it.

A mixture of fright and pain is a very distressing emotional experience. Small children often cry after a minor bump, not so much because of the pain, but in response to the pain plus anxiety transmitted by the mother as she rushes to comfort the child. In a sense, the child learns that it should be upset by the event, and once upset probably feels the pain more acutely. Children who are approached calmly and handled with the minimum of fuss and fright after a minor injury usually go on to cope calmly themselves in later life. Those for whom each small accident has become a major trauma, tend to go on reacting in an over-emotional way, and may also feel pain more intensely.

In good health care management, the team will seek to reassure and inform patients during procedures where pain might occur. They will know that a calm and confident patient will cope with the procedure better, and be able to co-operate, whereas someone anxious and anticipating discomfort will be harder to help, and will experience more distress and more pain. Attaining that state of calmness and confidence is in everyone's best interest. A relaxed state of mind is the first prerequisite for successful pain management.

Another important aspect of the mental state in pain experience is the sense of being in control. In hospital burns units, patients who are able to may be allowed to help with their own dressing changes and debridement. Debridement is the removal of damaged flesh and can cause great pain. Those for whom this option is open have shown far less distress, and complained of less pain, than those who must lie there helpless while these things are done to them. Patients have also been known to conspire, keeping their own outward expressions of pain and discomfort as minimal as they can in order to calm and reassure those coming new into the ward. Stories such as this tell us in no uncertain terms how well people understand the roles of fear, and of calmness and control, in pain.

Other beneficial results have been obtained in necessary but painful procedures when the patient is allowed to direct the pace at which things are done, or to assist in such things as handling equipment. This sense of being in control, of being a useful part of the proceedings, is also a major part of the success of natural childbirth techniques. There women are encouraged to manage aspects of labour rather than undergo it passively. They may choose to walk around between contractions; to use breathing techniques during contractions; and, if they want to, to give birth in a squatting or sitting up position and to help with the delivery. Pain is likely to be experienced as far less intense in these situations than in those where the person is required to lie flat and do nothing. A sense of helplessness enhances pain; a sense of control diminishes it.

In addition to calmness and a sense of being in control, another mental attribute important in pain management is the ability to focus the attention on something, and sustain that focusing so that the awareness of other things is diminished. We all do this all the time, of course. We can become so engrossed by a good book, or music, or a creative hobby, or a gripping story someone is telling us that we lose track of time and events going on round us. We can, consciously and at will, let one thing dominate the whole of our attention, so that other things cannot impinge, including pain. The extreme examples of this are the religious ecstatics, who are able to have hooks and knives put through their flesh, or to walk on hot coals, or to undergo hours of tortuous physical postures, and remain serene and free from pain. Fortunately, we do not need to go to those extremes in order to learn some control over pain. The deeply, totally absorbed attention required is something familiar to most of us; it simply needs applying. We need to turn it on when necessary, rather than just to let it happen by chance.

Although pain often fixes our attention on itself, and can become a more and more dominant part of our lives, this need not be so. Someone alone and in pain, even from a minor wound or headache, may feel unable to concentrate on anything but the pain, but the appearance of a welcome visitor may distract the sufferer, who then finds that the pain has gone. This is a very common experience. Attention-switching or distraction is not always easy to achieve by design at first, but it can be learned and used in pain control.

Finally, our attitude to pain is important. The meaning we give to pain can have a powerful effect for good or bad. If it is regarded as a frightening, little-understood threat to health, way of life or even life itself, it will become imbued with feelings of panic. A combination of pain and fear can be powerfully destructive, as each makes the other more intense. In this state, the autonomic nervous system is 'aroused' (that is, it is preparing the body to respond to threat by increasing cardiac rate and output, blood-pressure, respiration, blood supply to the muscles and skin, and metabolic rate). However, pain and fear cannot be evaded by running away, or conquered by a physical fight. Indeed, the aroused state can only make things worse, and is also likely to inhibit the ability to think and plan logically. It is vitally important then to know and understand the pain, so that ignorance of what is happening cannot generate panic.

The essential factors in psychological pain control then are understanding, mental calmness, physical relaxation, and the ability to focus the attention on something other than the pain, and hold it there. There is nothing strange or mystical about any of these attributes. They are all natural states and are common to us all. The only trick involved is to be able to turn them on consciously, rather than waiting and hoping for them to happen. That 'trick' can be learnt. Moreover, there is no one fixed way of turning on the necessary states; there are numerous variations which can be tailor-made for the individual. Once you have learnt the basics, you can design your own programme. It should be emphasized, however, that it is a process of learning. No one can learn a significant skill in five minutes; it must be worked at. The skill is comparable to playing the violin. Once someone has shown you how to hold the instrument and slide the bow across the strings, you will be able to make a noise. To play Bach, however, needs relaxed, focused attention and control applied over time. To achieve effective pain control, we need to aim for Bach.

Another point worth emphasizing is that this approach is not the same as that advocated by those who will have us believe that we can abolish pain by adopting the right attitude and thinking beautiful thoughts. Far from it. It would be wonderful if pain could be switched off by the magic power of the mind, but we know that it cannot. It is insulting to anyone in severe chronic pain to suggest that their thinking is all that is wrong.

The psychological methods described here are based on learning, and their purpose is to minimize or abolish those aspects of the pain attributable to fear, tension and focusing on the pain. When these are out of the way, there is a new perspective on the problem. The pain will be felt less acutely and will cease to be a dominant feature in the life of the victim. In addition, that person will know that they have effected the change. They are now in control, and are free from the tyranny of the pain. In some cases, they will then be able to become so absorbed in other things that the pain will indeed be abolished, for periods of time or completely. In others, the perspective will change, the freedom from tyranny will be achieved, mood and the quality of life will be enhanced, and the pain will still be there. Tucked away in a corner perhaps, but still there.

8. Relaxation Techniques in Pain Control

Pain is a source of stress, and stress has wide-ranging effects on the body, on feeling, thinking and behaviour. In situations where the pain has no function, none of these effects is helpful. On the contrary, they tend to make the experience of pain worse.

First, the pain can cause physiological arousal, so that the heart beat becomes faster and stronger, breathing becomes rapid, blood tends to flow away from the deep organs into the muscles and skin, and the body is at 'alert'. This is characteristically accompanied by an increase in muscle tension. Increased tension may affect all the muscles, but it can be particularly marked around the pain site. Instinctively, we 'guard' the painful part of the body, as if holding it very still will stop further damage. In non-functional pain all this does is to produce more pain from the tense muscles. We may fear that to relax the muscles will increase the pain; the reverse is true.

In addition to the body's arousal and the tensing of muscles, pain also tends to produce feelings of distress and anxiety. In acute types of pain these feelings may have a use — they generate a sense of urgency so that we do something about the pain-producing situation. In non-functional pain, they merely add another unpleasant dimension to the already unpleasant sensation of pain.

In this state of arousal and distress we tend not to be able to think clearly and logically, and may be unable to form sensible plans to help ourselves.

Pain changes our behaviour. Strong pain may cause us to walk about restlessly, or to thrash about on the bed. These are not useful pieces of behaviour and may make the pain seem stronger.

Learning to relax into pain is not easy when we seem under the control of these 'instincts'. However, it is important to remember that arousal, tension, distress and restlessness have no place in the management of non-injurious pain; they might be useful to prime us to run away from something hurting us, but pain of the type we are concerned with cannot be escaped from by running. It needs taking in hand.

As a first step in relaxing try this simple exercise. You can do it standing, sitting, or lying down — choose the most comfortable posture. Now put your hands just under your ribcage in front.

Now breathe in steadily and evenly to the count of three. Hold your breath briefly, then breathe out again to the count of three. Get an easy rhythm going — in, two, three, hold, out, two, three. In, two, three, hold, out, two, three. Keep the pace steady, and do not try to breathe extra deeply. Notice how your hands are gently pushed out and down on the outbreaths and in and up on the inbreaths. Keep the touch of your hands light. As you go on with the even, steady rhythm, 'let go' and relax a little more with each outbreath. Breathe in the good, cool air and breathe a sense of calm in with it. Breathe out the stale air and let the tension go with it. After only a minute or so you will feel different; calmer and more in control. You can do this exercise anywhere. In public you could do it without putting your hands over your diaphragm and no one would notice what you were doing. It is a quick, easy method of relaxation, and you may find it sufficient on its own to give you some pain control.

Where muscles are particularly tense, however, you may need to dispel that tension in a more systematic way, by working on one muscle group after another, all over the body. This technique, called progressive muscular relaxation, was pioneered by Edmund Jacobson, and it has been successfully adapted by pain therapists and others as a treatment for a variety of ailments, including psychosomatic problems and various painful conditions. First, minimize any distractions. Make sure the light is not in your eyes. Find a quiet place, and pick a time when you are unlikely to be disturbed for twenty minutes or so. Take off your shoes and loosen any tight clothing like ties, waistbands or belts. Then get comfortable. Find an armchair which supports your arms, back and head without strain, or lie down on a bed or sofa. Make sure you are *really* comfortable — nothing sticking into you, no hard places, nothing distorting your posture or pushing you into an awkward position.

Now focus your attention on your breathing. Breathe steadily in the pattern described above for ten to fifteen breaths. Then let your attention focus on your forehead and face. Slowly raise your eyebrows as far as you can, and feel the tension building up in your forehead and around your eyes. Now relax the muscles you have just used in pushing your eyebrows up, and notice how pleasant it feels to relax after the tension. Next, close your eyes then screw them up tight. This time the tension will be increased around your eyes and nose. It is uncomfortable. Let it go, and relax back to a normal position. Again, notice the pleasant feeling of relief and release as you do so. Now stretch your mouth in a 'grin' as far as you can, keeping your teeth together. Then relax. Now push your bottom jaw out so that the bottom teeth are in front of the top teeth. Notice how the tension builds in your lower face and chin. Now relax. Notice how your face feels with all the tension drained away from it.

Now think about the base of your head and your neck and shoulders. Slowly, without snatching at the muscles, bring your shoulders up in a shrug. Notice carefully where the tension and discomfort have their effect. Now relax and let your shoulders slowly return to an easy resting position. Next, turn your head round to the left and feel the tension building in the right side of your neck and right shoulder. Then let your head slowly come back to face front. Repeat the exercise, turning your head to the right this time. Remember that all these exercises must be carried out slowly, smoothly and gently.

Now lift your arms up until they are level with your shoulders and gradually stretch them away from you. Stretch all along your arms into your elbows, wrists and fingers — spread the fingers well out. Then relax and let your arms slowly drift down to your sides again. Then, to get any remaining tension out of your hands, slowly screw them up into fists. Hold tight like that, and then relax again.

Next, your back. Keeping your shoulders and bottom where they are, arch the middle of your back into an inward curve. Hold that position briefly, then relax again.

Now pull in the muscles of your abdomen so that you feel as firm and flat as you can. Hold it, then relax.

Next, pull in the muscles in your bottom, hold that position briefly, then relax again.

Now your legs. Stretch them out away from your body until you can feel the stiffness and tension all the way down into your feet. Then relax and let them rest.

Finally, pull your toes towards you, then relax; screw them up under your feet (gently!) and relax again.

Now check all over your body and re-tense and relax any part of you still feeling 'tight'. When you are fully relaxed you may feel lighter, as if you could float away, or you may feel heavier, as if you could sink down through the bed; reactions vary. In either case, just let yourself go with the feeling. Sink down, down into deeper relaxation if you want to, or float peacefully into an ever-more-relaxed state.

There are two golden rules for this kind of progressive relaxation:
1. Make each movement in a slow and carefully controlled way. Never 'snatch' at the muscles when you tense, and never let go suddenly when you relax. Gently does it.
2. If it hurts, leave it out! For some people with muscular problems, especially in the neck or back, tensing the muscles, even gently, may hurt. In these cases, leave out the tensing part of the sequence and, when you get to that group of muscles, just let them relax. It should all be a pleasant, soothing experience.

Emotional effects

Many people feel an immediate sense of well-being and contentment when they relax like this for the first time. For some, however, the release of the tension is accompanied by weeping, usually on the first occasion. If this should happen, don't be alarmed. Weep all you need to. It is all part of the release of accumulated tension, and is not harmful. If it goes on happening every time you relax, do not persist with this technique. This is very unlikely to happen unless you are significantly depressed and have only been covering it up by being over-controlled. In such a case, seek help for the depression as a problem in its own right.

Sometimes, when you begin to relax for the first time, the opposite happens and an overwhelming desire to giggle takes over. Again, this is nothing to worry about. Let it happen. It usually occurs because there is some anxiety about 'letting go' and giggling is a defensive reaction. It does not usually persist beyond the first time. Enjoy it, then carry on with the technique once it has passed.

When you have been relaxing, even if you feel you have only been partly successful, it is very likely that your heart-rate, breathing and blood-pressure will be reduced. Remember to give your body time to adjust afterwards. Move your limbs around a little, stretch, and if you have been lying flat, put your feet down first and your head up last. Suddenly jumping up without this brief time of adaptation may make you feel dizzy or sick as your body makes a frantic effort to cope with a sudden demand for action.

In the long term
You will need to practise this once a day (twice if you can manage it) for about fifteen to twenty minutes. Most people feel a beneficial change the very first time, but it is usually only for a brief time. Continuing practice for four to six weeks gives a good, long-lasting result in which muscle tension is reduced and the body and mind should become calmer. In addition, you will, if successful, become 'tuned in' to your body so that you will be aware of the build-up of tension as soon as it starts. After the initial practice period, you may like to go on with a regular regime, or to use it when needed. Tailor-make it to suit your needs.

When you relax like that, you have taken control, become calm, and focused your attention — all the ingredients needed for the psychological management of pain. All the techniques described on the following pages have the same basic things underlying them; relaxation, focused attention, and control. Different techniques will be described because it is important to find your own way. DIFFERENT METHODS SUIT DIFFERENT PEOPLE. Not everyone will be able to use progressive muscular relaxation. Of those who can, it may not suit them all. Some people need the physical exercise dimension, others fare better with mental exercises. An essential part of taking control of your pain is making decisions about what you will do. You may try relaxation and find that it alone gives you pain control. Many people have done so. You may find that you need relaxation plus a meditative technique; you may prefer to meditate or use visual imagery only; you may get most benefit from self-hypnosis (autogenic training) with no specific physical movements. It is for you to try the technique you feel will suit you best, and practise until you perfect it, modifying it if necessary to give you the best results. Research has tended to show closely similar physiological changes in progressive muscular relaxation, hypnosis and meditation. All have been shown to be beneficial to health, and successful in regimes of stress management and pain control. It is for you to decide on the recipe and use it.

9. Autogenic Training

Hypnosis has long been successfully used to treat pain. Many dentists now use it for pain control; it is used in some burns units during painful procedures and even in some casualty departments when wounds are being stitched. There are many examples of its use in the treatment of pain.

What is hypnosis?

We may tend to think that there are two states of mind common to us: consciousness, when we are awake, and unconsciousness, when we are asleep. However, some further thought will reveal that it is not as simple as that. Any one who has had a young baby, or a sick child or elderly relative in the house, will know that during sleep we are not always unconscious. We may appear to be so, but be woken by the slightest sound from the one we feel anxious about. We may sleep through loud noises, like traffic passing outside, but be instantly roused by someone turning over restlessly in bed in another room. While we sleep, our brains are actively receiving information and sorting it so that we can respond selectively. A very striking example of this was given by a mother whose small baby was admitted to hospital as an emergency. The mother went too and was given a bed in the baby's room. She was exhausted by worry over the child and went to sleep early. The child stirred around in his cot at 10 p.m. and 2 a.m., and she woke, fed and changed him. The nurses thought the baby must have slept all through the night as they had heard no noise at all; he had not cried; his mother had responded to his restless movements. During the night, the nurses had come into the room three times to carry out observations on the baby. This necessitated their walking past the mother's bed. She had not stirred, and in the morning they teased her about how deeply she had been sleeping.

Even in sleep we are actively monitoring some aspects of our environment and responding to them at different levels of consciousness.

If this happens in sleep, this multi-layered consciousness, then it is even more striking in the waking state. We find ourselves upstairs, or in the kitchen, and suddenly 'come to' wondering why we are there. We came there purposefully, as if for a good reason, but it has slipped into another layer of our consciousness and for the moment we cannot recall it. It will surface again later. We may listen to someone talking, and respond appropriately, but then cannot remember a word of what was said because the mind was 'elsewhere'. Sometimes in a room full of people talking, we suddenly become aware that someone has been trying to attract our attention and we respond with 'sorry — I was miles away' or even 'sorry — I was in a trance'. There are numerous other examples in daily life of the fact that we can slip in and out between coexisting layers of consciousness quite naturally. The hypnotic state is an example of this. It is a natural state, familiar to most of us. In hypnosis there is usually a guide (hypnotist or hypnotherapist) who aids the process, but all hypnosis is essentially self-hypnosis. The subject elects to enter the state, rather than waiting for it to happen by chance, and the hypnotist assists, or helps to induce the trance.

Once in the trance state, we find it easier to do certain things than when we are in an habitual fully-alert state of consciousness with all its busyness and distractions. The capacity to imagine and fantasize is greatly enhanced, as is the ability of the mind to influence certain things about the body, in a very strong and striking way. Anaesthesia can be produced, for example, completely enough for lesions to be made or pins pushed through the skin and no pain to be felt. Suggestions of warmth or cold in parts of the body can result in observable and measurable changes in temperature. Pain from an organic source such as a wound or disease process can be blocked. Physical stillness and deep, focused inner calm seem to be the key.

The self-induced trance

Eighty or so years ago, some subjects taking part in a series of experiments on sleep and hypnosis told researchers that they had been putting themselves into the hypnotic state between experiments, and using it to control tension and stress, and to abolish stress-related headaches and other similar symptoms. This formed the basis of autogenic (that is, self-induced) hypnosis training, which was developed into a standard technique by Luthe and others from 1960 on.

Studies have shown that when people practise the technique over a period of time, most of them report feeling more relaxed and confident, and apart from feeling generally better, many have been specifically helped with problems like migraine, irritable bowel, insomnia, and high blood-pressure.

Like progressive muscular relaxation (p.m.r.), autogenic training begins with getting comfortable on a bed, sofa, armchair or cushions on the floor. Some trainers advise taking up weird postures, such as kneeling on the floor, leaning forward with the forehead against a stool or chair seat; or sitting on a chair, leaning forward, with the forearms across the thighs, hands dangling between the thighs. It is difficult to see what possible advantage could be gained from such contortions, and they are best avoided, especially by anyone with neck, shoulder or back pain. Comfort is the most important thing.

When you are really comfortable, with nothing pushing or twisting your body or causing any tension in your posture, focus on your breathing. Do not take great deep breaths, but concentrate on breathing in feelings of calmness, and relaxing on each outbreath, as in p.m.r. Allow yourself to 'let go' as you breathe steadily and easily in and out. After a minute or so, let your attention turn to any tense or painful parts of your body, one at a time. Do not try to change anything; merely direct your attention to the area of discomfort and explore it. Notice exactly what it feels like, but make no attempt to analyze it. Notice it, carefully and unemotionally, and then let it be.

Now you are going to let yourself go into trance by letting one part of your body after another become loose, warm and heavy. You do this by repeating the following 'trigger' phrases to yourself silently, taking your time, with plenty of pauses in between, as you direct your attention to each part. Go on until you feel the effect you want, then move on to the next part of your body. Here is the sequence:

My right arm is feeling heavy
My right arm is feeling heavier
My right arm is heavy

My left arm is feeling heavy
My left arm is feeling heavier
My left arm is heavy

My right arm is becoming warm
My right arm is becoming warmer
My right arm is warm

My left arm is becoming warm
My left arm is becoming warmer
My left arm is warm

My right leg is feeling heavy
My right leg is feeling heavier
My right leg is heavy

My left leg is feeling heavy
My left leg is feeling heavier
My left leg is heavy

My right leg is feeling warm
My right leg is feeling warmer
My right leg is warm

My left leg is feeling warm
My left leg is feeling warmer
My left leg is warm

As these feelings of warmth and heaviness develop and steal over the limbs, the body becomes quieter and quieter and more and more deeply relaxed, and the mind slips into the trance state. Now go on with the final parts of the induction, again repeating them slowly to yourself until the effect develops:

My heart beat is calm and regular
My breathing is calm and regular
My forehead is cool and light
I am at peace with myself and fully relaxed

You may be lucky enough to achieve the trance state the first time you try, but it is more likely that you will get fleeting experiences of 'letting go' at first. You will need to persevere in order to deepen and lengthen those experiences until you remain in trance for as long as you want to. Daily practice is best to begin with, until you can reliably attain the desired state. You should find that the induction becomes easier and quicker as time goes on.

When you want to come out of the trance state, you can simply count backwards from five to one, like countdown to take-off. As you count, let yourself come up out of the trance fully awake and alert by the count of one. As with p.m.r., give yourself time to adjust briefly before you get up. Stretch your limbs, or move them around gently, as you might when waking from sleep. Remember that your blood-pressure will probably have dropped and your heart-rate and breathing will be slow, so do not jump up quickly or you may feel faint or giddy.

Once in the trance state you can use a variety of imaginal devices and suggestions for pain control. Before you begin, prepare yourself by thinking about what eases your pain and building an imaginary scene around it, to use in the trance state. If, for example, you find that warmth usually eases the pain, you might go into trance and then imagine you are under a sun lamp with the lamp focused on the painful part of your body. Turn on the lamp and feel the healing rays on your skin. Slowly the area the lamp is shining on becomes warmer, and as it does so the pain begins to ease and to fade. The warm, gentle rays are doing their work and taking the pain away. Notice how good it feels to have warmth in that area. Let the lamp shine on until all the pain has gone. Then, even when you turn the lamp off, you will go on feeling warmth for some while. Cover the skin up to hold the warmth in so that the freedom from pain continues. The pain-free time will gradually extend beyond the trance as time goes on and you become more skilled. The sun lamp scene is, of course, only one example. You might like to use an image of the sun itself, shining on a tropical beach while you laze in a deckchair; or of warm water on your skin; or a warm, soft piece of cloth being bound round the painful part.

If coolness is what helps the pain, you might imagine a scene where an ice pack is being applied to the affected part, and slowly the coldness creeps into your skin numbing it and taking away the pain as it does so. Or perhaps a fountain or waterfall could be playing on your body. Feel the tingle of the water; listen to it, and feel that part of your body getting cooler as the water takes the pain away.

Perhaps nothing simple eases your pain, but you lose it as you drift into sleep. You can recreate that too. You can let yourself drift into sleep, imagining that you are in a very cosy bed which is warm and slowly lulling you to sleep. Feel the pain drifting away as your mind and body relax into sleep. Let yourself drift down, down, down. Remember, though, to set a clock or timer for when you want to wake!

Each time you use one of these devices, tell yourself that when you come out of trance the pain will still be removed from you.

If you are successful, you could attain long periods of pain control in this way. First, however, you must become skilled at going into trance and bringing yourself out, and also at deepening the trance. You may be able to do this by just letting yourself go each time you breathe out, once you have gone into the trance, for about ten breaths. You could try counting yourself down. You could try imagining yourself going slowly down some steps or down in a lift until you are at the level you want to be. You will probably need to deepen the trance to get effective pain control. At the end of the time you want to spend in the trance, come back up in the lift, or up the stairs, or count yourself up, or come up with each breath. Take time to perfect your autogenic skills; you may be disappointed in the results if you fail to do the groundwork properly.

Before you embark on autogenic training, talk it over with your doctor or someone else who knows about autogenics. Although it is perfectly safe for most people, there are some forms of psychological disturbance and some forms of epilepsy which may be exacerbated by the trance state. It might also cause emotional upset in some people. If you cry at first, it may just be the relief at letting go, but if that weeping is accompanied by distressing thoughts or feelings, you could be uncovering something you need help with, and you should seek professional help. You might like to start working with a trainer rather than alone.

Autogenic training is increasingly available. Some health centres provide it; ask your GP. Or you could write to the Centre for Autogenic Training, 101 Harley Street, London, W1N 1DF (send a s.a.e.) for a list of qualified teachers working in the private sector.

10. Meditation

Progressive muscular relaxation (p.m.r.) produces physiological changes in the body. Heart rate, respiration rate, blood-pressure and muscle tone are all reduced during relaxation. Autogenic training produces similar results. The difference in the two approaches is that progressive relaxation uses muscular movements *and* focused attention, while autogenic training is a purely mental or inner technique. Calmness and focused attention can have profound effects on the body. Meditation, in any of its forms, is a technique for attention-focusing and can have a powerful effect on the body too.

Within the broad term 'meditation' there are very many variations, but they have in common the idea of channelling the mind's activity away from its usual busy, discursive, logical/analytical concerns and focusing on something which produces a deep inner peace. The use of meditation stretches back beyond written history, and may be as old as man himself. It has featured in many religions, from Buddha's teaching to both early and modern Christianity. In the religious life, meditation may bring not only a sense of deep peace, but also spiritual enlightenment. Terms such as 'attaining Nirvana', 'cosmic awareness', 'the still deep centre of the self', or 'reaching God', are used to describe the desired state. It is, then, obviously a profound and moving experience, with qualities markedly different from ordinary thought.

Bodily changes during meditation
Research has shown that all the physiological responses produced by p.m.r. and autogenic training can also be produced by meditation. The body goes into a state similar to that found on the borders of sleep, but the mind is not asleep. It is a paradoxical state sometimes described as alert-yet-deeply-resting. Again, this

state is common to p.m.r., autogenic training and meditation. The means to attain it differ, but the end result is similar. The regular practice of any of them is beneficial to health and an important part of stress-control and anxiety management. Pain is a stressor. Pain and external sources of stress are closely related, in that they produce similar patterns of change in the body, in the self, and in behaviour. It follows that similar management regimes could be used for pain and stress. All these techniques also have in common the fact that regular practice is the key to success. In this respect, some forms of meditation have the edge on the other techniques, as they are part of a cult or pattern of beliefs, and membership of the cult gives a sense of identity with the group. Commitment to a group and its ideals, and a sense of belonging to something good and powerful, may help to keep people meditating when they might have given up on a similar technique with no such background. It depends on your needs, and the type of person you are. Since Transcendental Meditation has an almost world-wide following, with millions of devotees, it seems that the sense of belonging and the group support fill a basic need for many of us. Others will be put off by the quasi-religious nature of the belief system. Transcendental Meditation (T.M.) is one variation of mantra meditation which will be described here, as will object meditation. There are many variations on the basic idea — too many to describe here in detail, but the examples used will give a general idea of how to go about meditating.

Mantra meditation
There is some controversy about the use of mantras, or words, in meditation. Some people believe that the 'wrong' mantra can be harmful. In T.M., for example, each new meditator is given a personal mantra by a teacher, and the mantras are chosen to suit the individual. That is not to say that everyone has a uniquely different mantra; they are chosen to suit the broad circumstances of the meditator, so that there are certain mantras for the young, certain mantras for those who lead retiring lives, others for those who are out in the world. In T.M. mantras are Sanskrit words which have no meaning in themselves, so they cannot produce distracting associations. That is the theory, although the fertile human brain can in fact produce associations to most things, whether or not they have a denotative meaning. Mantras might be words like 'shirrim' or 'aum'. Some research has also been carried out using meaningful words like sky and love (positive) or hate

(negative). Most people taking part found that the positive words made them feel good, and negative words made them feel bad, but there were some odd people who preferred the negative words . . .

Perhaps the lesson to be learnt from all this is find a word that suits you. Try a likely neutral, meaningless or positive word to meditate with. If it makes you physically deeply relaxed, and mentally deeply calm, and you feel good afterwards, stick with it. If you cannot settle physically while you are using it, and your thoughts stray into dark and miserable by-ways, and you feel heavy or sad afterwards, change it.

First, as in all the techniques, get comfortable. Sit in an easy chair or on the floor, in a restful posture. Make sure the room you are in is quiet, airy, and neither too hot nor too cold. Try to choose a time when you are unlikely to be disturbed, or make it known that you do not wish to be disturbed for at least fifteen minutes. Loosen tight clothing, and get rid of any distractions. Now begin to repeat your chosen word to yourself, silently. Take your time. Listen to the sound the word makes in your mind but do not try to analyse it or think about it. Just go on repeating it to yourself. If your mind wanders, do not worry. This will happen to begin with. Let it finish the wandering, and then go on repeating the mantra. As you go on, your attention will be drawn inwards and downwards, to the quiet depths of the mind. Wakeful awareness will slowly give way to a state in which the mind is deeply calm and still, and yet is not asleep. Awareness will be heightened, but contained within. Each time you meditate, at the beginning, you will get better and faster at reaching the desired state of inner calm. Fifteen minutes' practice, once a day (or better still twice, morning and evening) will produce a healthful rest for your mind and body. Experienced meditators tend to recover faster from stressful stimuli than non-meditators, and also to show signs of relaxed, absorbed attention on EEG (brainwave) measurement for periods when they are not meditating. The effects of habitual meditation go beyond the time spent in meditation, and produce learned changes in reaction which are important in stress control, and therefore in pain control.

Object meditation
Some people are visualizers. They can conjure up pictures in their 'mind's eye', and they tend to use and enjoy visual images. If you are a visualizer, using mantra meditation may or may not appeal

to you. If it does not, or you find it particularly hard to use a word with no images associated with it, perhaps object meditation is better for you. You can use a real or imagined object. Find something with pleasant associations — a rose, a leaf, a pebble or seashell, a piece of beautiful fabric, the flame of a candle, a pleasing piece of pottery or sculpture. First, as ever, get comfortable and relax. Breathe steadily and easily for a minute or two, and then begin to contemplate your chosen object. A red rose will serve as an example. To begin with, you might turn your attention to the colour. Absorb the deep redness, and let it absorb you. Do not try to make conscious associations or judgements, simply let the red colour take you into it, like a soft enveloping cloud. As the deep redness spreads round you, begin to be aware of the fragrance of the rose. Breathe in the essence of the rose, gently and slowly, over and over again. Deep redness all around you, sweet fragrance within. Hold on to that as long as you can, and then let your attention also take in the texture of the petals. Soft, smooth and velvety. Imagine the velvetiness on your fingertips, then let all your fingers slide across the petals, then your whole hand. Slowly, let the soft velvet feeling spread to your arms and shoulders, over your neck and face, over your whole body. The colour, scent and feel of the rose have enveloped and absorbed you. You are the rose, and it is you. Stay with it as long as you want to or need to, then, slowly pull back and away.

These few words will give some idea of what you can aim at in object meditation. As with mantra meditation, it will probably take practice for you to be able to attain a degree of relaxed, absorbed attention so profound that you become absorbed totally in your object, and are thus detached from your body and its concerns, including your pain.

At first, your attention will inevitably wander, and you may attain the desired state in frustratingly brief periods only. Do not be concerned about it. It is a skill like any other; your performance will be halting and imperfect to start with, but it will improve over time and with practice.

The use of music

Music can be a powerful aid to meditation. It is a question of personal choice and preference. If you are someone who likes music, and someone for whom music can evoke or sustain a certain mood, you might like to try it in meditation. Choose something peaceful and beautiful, and reasonably long, so that you can sustain the meditative state for several minutes as you get more skilled. As with mantra and object meditation, the object is to attend with total absorption, but uncritically. It is important to set the volume at a comfortable level, not so soft that you are straining to hear the quieter passages, and not so loud as to be overwhelming. The basic technique is the same as in the other forms of meditation, to be relaxed and comfortable, and then to let the music take you into itself. You may find that it produces a series of images in your mind, or that your mind remains quiet, and the sound is all. It does not matter which. It is simply a question of letting go, and going where the music takes you.

One most important ingredient in the successful practice of meditation is to find what suits you. First of all, be guided by what feels right for you. You are the best judge of whether mantra, object or music is best for you, or perhaps some other variation not described here. You are likely to be most successful with something which feels comfortable for you. Secondly, be guided by the effect the meditation has on you. It should make you feel well, strong, and at peace. If after meditating you feel heavy, gloomy or unwell, try an alternative form of meditation or another technique altogether. As with autogenic training, take medical advice before you begin, as meditation may be detrimental for people with some kinds of psychological illness or some forms of epilepsy.

11. Visual Imagery

Some forms of visual imagery have already been described in the chapters on autogenic training and meditation. Creating a peaceful scene in the mind's eye is also often used after the gentle physical exercises in p.m.r. to deepen the relaxation and help to quieten the mind. However, this chapter will be concerned with a particular form of visual imagery, which is being increasingly used in healing, notably with cancer patients, and with some kinds of hypnotherapy. In this form of visual imagery, a pictorial representation of the problem is formed in the mind, and it is resolved in the mind. For example, her racing pulse was represented by one patient as a pump which was working too fast. When she had clearly envisaged the pump, she added a large knob to the image, which could be slowly adjusted to decrease the rate of pumping. A cancer patient saw her tumour as like a 'lump of horrible hamburger meat' and she conjured up legions of hungry white blood cells which were gobbling up the horrible hamburger little by little. Yet another patient with high blood-pressure saw it as like a boiler with too much pressure, on which he would open a safety valve and let some steam out until the pressure gradually dropped. Of course, simply thinking about these things is not enough. They need to be carried out as mental or inner exercises after p.m.r. or autogenic training has produced a significant degree of physiological quieting.

The value of visual imagery
What is the value of visual imagery? As yet there is no scientific research on it. All we have so far is enthusiasm about its beneficial effects from small numbers of patients. Autogenics, p.m.r. and meditation have all been studied, and the results of the research tend to show two things:
1. Measurable changes in blood-pressure, heart rate, respiration

rate and EEG (the recording of electrical activity from the brain). These changes are in the direction of physiological quieting in the body, coupled with an alert picture from the EEG, showing the alert-yet-deeply-resting or relaxed absorbed attention pattern. Regular practice produces long-term effects such as less reactivity and quicker recovery from stress, and several studies have shown that the risk of heart attack can be significantly reduced by the practice of one or other regime, and long lasting reductions in high blood-pressure have been shown. Conditions with pain as a major factor, such as back problems, muscular-skeletal pain, some forms of migraine and other headaches, have also been helped by regular relaxation regimes, with reports of fewer episodes of pain and less need for pain-killers. These are long-term effects.

2. Many practitioners report enhanced well-being and reductions in nervous and psychosomatic disorders, often with freedom from dependence on tranquillizers after many years. Some GP health centres are now offering autogenic training classes, and at least one GP recommends meditation to many of her patients for conditions like insomnia, irritable bowel and headache, and smoking, alcohol or tranquillizer dependence.

It is clear then that there are powerful positive effects from a variety of relaxation regimes. Relaxation techniques are also regularly taught to patients (inpatients and outpatients) seeking help with pain control from pain clinics up and down the country. In these cases the source of the pain may be anything from scars to back pain to cancer, or perhaps one of the puzzling chronic pains mentioned earlier. The type and source of pain is immaterial. The fact is that a proportion of patients, even with far-advanced cancer, have been successful in controlling pain using these techniques. The cornerstone to all of them seems to be the capacity for relaxed absorbed attention, developed to a high degree of skill. Why visual imagery rather than any other technique?

There may be nothing to recommend visual imagery as superior to the other techniques, except that it is preferred by some people and felt by them to be more beneficial. It is, in a way, a more direct attempt to be in touch with the body and its disorders than other meditative techniques. For many people it gives an enhanced feeling of being in control of what is going on inside them, and is more relevant than a mantra or the image of a rose. As it is investigated, it may turn out to be a superior technique to the others or it may not. At present the enthusiasm of those who have used it successfully is its main recommendation, and as it is part of a relaxation regime, it will have all the benefits known to come from them. These are good enough reasons to include it here for those who feel it is the right method for them.

How to use visual imagery

First of all, you will need to think carefully and calmly about your pain, and to explore its precise nature. What is it like? Is it a dull ache, a sharp twinge, a deep throb? Writing down a few adjectives might help. How big an area of your body is affected by the pain? How deep? Does it have a certain shape? Is it dense or spongey? Does it make the affected part feel heavy, hot, brittle, taut? How does it make you feel?

All these things are a necessary part of forming a clear image of the pain for yourself. Next, perhaps you could try to draw a representation of it.

When you have successfully explored your pain and formed a picture of it, the next step is to decide what to change. If, for example, you see the pain as a sharp needle sticking into you, something slowly pulling it out might help. Something blunting or covering the end of it might help. Fluid bathing the tissues round it might help. If you see the pain as a tight band, a device for loosening it will be needed. A hot, tense pain might need ice or a cool bath. It is for you to imagine an effective remedy.

When you have the picture of the pain and its remedy clear in your mind, the next step is to learn and perfect one of the quieting techniques described here. You might choose p.m.r., autogenics or meditation, whichever you find to be most effective. You will need to become skilled enough to quieten your body to the point where you are scarcely aware of it, and to attain a stillness in the mind like the state between the borders of sleeping and waking: a trance state. When you can get into this state readily and consistently, let your attention turn to the painful part of your body and 'see' the pain as you have prepared yourself to. Allow a good strong image to develop and then introduce your remedy to the fantasy. Take it slowly and do not try to achieve everything at once. Some successful dulling of the pain is better than a failed attempt to stop it altogether. Build on each small success time by time, day by day. Practise regularly and prepare yourself by quieting equally thoroughly each time.

Indirect imaging

You might find it easiest to 'see' your pain as a needle, an electric current, a screw, a rock, or something similar. Then you will need an appropriate remedy to act upon it. It does not matter what you fantasize as long as it matches your pain convincingly for you, as you need never share it with anyone if you do not wish to. Try to avoid making it all too complex, as you will need to visualize it clearly. Try also to avoid the temptation to produce a comical image as laughing is really a way of avoiding tackling the issue. Here is an example of an indirect image for period pains:

It is like having a broad, stretchy band around my abdomen, with sharp steel pieces inside it, pointing inwards and downwards. At the beginning I am aware of a slightly tight feeling around my lower back and abdomen, and then slowly the rubber tightens and the steel digs into my flesh, deeper and deeper. It frightens me, and as the pain peaks, I sob and sweat. After a while it passes, but I know it will come back. I have felt helpless, but now I am not, as when I feel the tight band I grow a fantasy pair of arms with large, strong hands and fingers. Strong but gentle. I slide the hands under the band, between it and my abdomen. The outer fingers rest on the top of my pelvis and the thumbs almost meet in the middle. As the band begins to tighten the powerful hands slowly push outwards, counteracting the pressure. It is hard work to make them push, but I can do it. I can pour strength into them to lift the tightening band away from me and stop the sharp steel digging in. As the tightness passes, the hands relax and gather strength for the next time. They are my hands. My strength defeats the pain.

Direct imaging

Some people might find indirect imaging too fanciful and distracting, but still want to use visual imagery. For them, perhaps, trying to make a mental picture of what the inside of the body really looks like is better. There are numerous 'atlases' and medical books with detailed coloured drawings, from whole complexes of organs down to individual nerve-endings and blood vessels. You would need to choose something appropriate to your pain. You might, for example, need a picture of an arthritic knee joint, or perhaps the walls of cranial blood vessels with stretch receptors in them which will signal 'pain' when the vessels dilate. Choose something appropriate with which you feel comfortable. Get the chosen image clear in your mind, so that you can call it up when you want to. Find out the appropriate body mechanism for combating the pain. It might be soothing fluids produced by the body to bathe the afflicted place. It might be the endorphins, the body's natural pain-killers produced by the nervous system. As with the indirect imaging, build a convincing and manageable sequence for yourself and use it regularly under deep relaxation.

Ego-building

Whichever method you use, remember that you are taking part in a bold experiment using only what comes from within yourself. It will be hard work. You may not always get it right, and there will be times, inevitably, when you are low or tired, or the pain is strong, particularly at the beginning. It is important to build in a formula to cope with this, as letting a session end in apparent failure is discouraging and depressing. You could, for example, give yourself and the pain scores out of ten. If the pain scores more than you on one occasion, offer it a return match when you are feeling stronger, and always give yourself support. We are all good at self-denigration and often only too ready to parade our faults and weaknesses before our own critical eyes. Try to break yourself of this if you are a culprit; it is destructive. Always end a session of quieting (with or without imagery), whether it went well or not so well, by giving yourself some supportive self-talk. Run through your good points. Remind yourself how well you cope with all kinds of problems. Find and address your personal source of help and comfort, whether that comes from within you or from your god. Your sense of your own worth is vitally important — nourish it. If you do not care for yourself, why should you try to manage your pain? You could just let it go on hurting you, why not?

Index

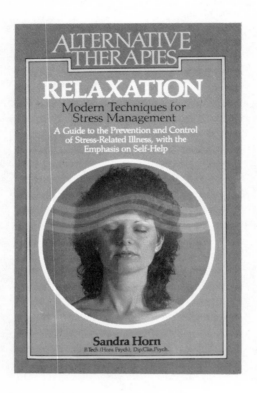

Of further interest

RELAXATION

Modern Techniques for Stress Management

'Stress' is a word we hear more and more often nowadays, yet it fails to convey the true depth of a problem that is far more than simply feeling upset or threatened. Stress can, and does, cause actual bodily changes that often result in very real physical or mental illness. **Sandra Horn** here explores the nature of stress, examines the varied ways in which different people react to it, and offers self-help management methods including: relaxation; biofeedback; transcendental meditation and other related techniques. *An excellent and informed self-help manual.*